preemie

LESSONS IN LOVE, LIFE AND MOTHERHOOD

preemie

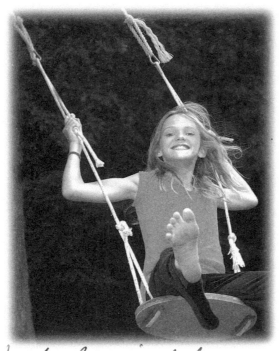

LESSONS IN LOVE, LIFE
AND MOTHERHOOD

KASEY MATHEWS

Hatherleigh Press is committed to preserving and protecting the natural
resources of the Earth. Environmentally responsible and sustainable
practices are embraced within the company's mission statement.

Hatherleigh Press is a member of the Publishers Earth Alliance, committed to preserving and protecting the natural resources of the planet while
developing a sustainable business model for the book publishing industry.

This book was edited and designed in the village of Hobart, New York.
Hobart is a community that has embraced books and publishing as a
component of its livelihood. There are several unique bookstores in the
village. For more information, please visit www.hobartbookvillage.com.

Library of Congress Cataloging-in-Publication Data is available
upon request.

ISBN 978-1-57826-423-0

Preemie is available for bulk purchase, special promotions, and premiums.
For information on reselling and special purchase opportunities, call
1-800-528-2550 and ask for the Special Sales Manager.

Cover and interior design by DCDESIGNS
Back cover photo by Shandy Welch
Photography on page 272 by Ramsay Thomas (www.mountainbliss.net)

10 9 8 7 6 5 4 3 2 1
Printed in the United States

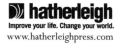

Improve your life. Change your world.
www.hatherleighpress.com

Advance Praise for *Preemie*

"In her enormously affecting memoir, Kasey Mathews writes with startling honesty about the emotional turmoil that engulfed her when her daughter Andie was born at 25 weeks, and the resulting guilt that followed Kasey for years thereafter. At its core, *Preemie* is a story about a mother emerging through her pain to find her strength and her voice—and ultimately finding herself in the process. *Preemie* is a tale that any mother going through personal challenges would find inspiring to read."

—*Sue L. Hall, M.D., Medical Director of the Neonatal Intensive Care Unit at Stormont-Vail HealthCare in Topeka, Kansas and author of* For the Love of Babies

"Just when you think you know nearly everything there is to know about what it feels like to be a human being, along comes a story that brings you to your knees and cracks your heart open just a bit more. *Preemie* is just that type of story. Kasey Mathews tells deep, painful truths about what happens when a 'perfect' life is jolted by reality. So much more than an account of a birth plan gone awry, this lovely memoir is about letting go of assumptions, moving into the place that scares us most, and discovering that what we get in return for our surrender is nothing less than grace."

—*Katrina Kenison, author of* The Gift of an Ordinary Day *and* Mitten Strings for God

"*Preemie* is an invaluable resource for families coping with the trauma of having a premature baby. Kasey Mathews elegantly and authentically describes her own preemie journey, becoming a best friend and mentor who has lived your experience and provides wisdom and tools that can help soothe and comfort you."

—*Libby Barnett, M.S.W., Reiki Master Teacher, author of* Reiki Energy Medicine

"*Preemie* is a frank, funny, touching, and triumphant story that will resonate with anyone who has loved a runt of any species, and deeply move everyone who has ever loved a baby of any kind."

—*Sy Montgomery, author of* The Good, Good Pig *and* Birdology

"*Preemie* is an inspiring story of love and courage."

—*Peggy Huddleston, author of* Prepare for Surgery, Heal Faster

"*Preemie* is a gripping tale of one mother's indefatigable love in the face of crisis, one baby's tenacious struggle to stay alive, and the dazzling light of self-exploration at the end of the tunnel. This tiny child will change the world."

—*Suzanne Kingsbury, author of* The Summer Fletcher Greel Loved Me *and* The Gospel According to Gracey

"Kasey Mathews speaks her true story with a voice as authentic as a newborn's cry. *Preemie* inspires us all to cherish and to share our own most harrowing adventures with humble courage."

—*Nancy Mellon, author of* Body Eloquence: The Power of Myth and Story to Awaken the Body's Energies

"The emotional, physical, financial, and psychological impact of having a child born pre-term often blindsides parents. *Preemie* captures the essence of life as the parent of a preemie. Kasey Mathews speaks with raw honesty about the fear, challenges, and emotional toll of mothering a medically fragile child. The book beautifully chronicles the transformational power of living through ones worst nightmare and coming out on the other side a fuller self. It is a must read for all parents of preemies and those who love them."

—*Kelli Kelley, mother of two preemies and Founder and Executive Director of Hand to Hold*

"The gift of *Preemie* is Kasey Mathews' ability to share her deepest feelings of fear, guilt, grief, anger, post-traumatic stress, humor, and joy. Her honesty with herself and others will be a wonderful companion for those who experience the challenging, life-changing experience of giving birth to a preemie. As Kasey deals with her raw emotions, she begins to 'attune' to the life force energy within herself and her daughter, Andie, and opens up to the wonderful healing energies all around her. With the unconditional love of her husband, Lee, and the protective love of big brother, Tucker, Kasey can step back and embrace her vision of her beautiful, healthy little girl. Love and light to this special family that will be a beacon of hope and empowerment to others."

— *Julie Hahn, Chaplain and Reiki Coordinator, Brigham and Women's Hospital*

"You don't have to have had a preemie to love this book. *Preemie* is a beautiful and intriguing memoir of Kasey Mathews' nightmarish experience bringing her daughter into the world. The writing is lovely, chronicling a journey none of us want to take, but one we know we would survive after reading Kasey's inspiring tale."

—*Bonnie Harris, author of* When Your Kids Push Your Buttons *and* Confident Parents, Remarkable Kids

"The emotions this book has made surface are beyond words. It helped me release many things I was not aware I have been carrying. With many spiritual teachers in my life, I am adding Kasey Mathews to the list."

—*Chick Wetherbee, Owner of Earthward Natural Foods and Co-op*

"*Preemie* teaches us the importance of finding your voice and stepping into your own authority, especially in times of personal crisis. Little Andie, the book's tiny heroine who boasts strength to spare, teaches us about persevering against all odds. Important lessons for us all!"

—*Tricia Rose Burt, writer and frequent guest storyteller*
on The Moth: True Stories Told Live

"A book you won't put down until you have read the very last word. *Preemie* is a beautifully written, moving account of a family's journey with their extremely early born daughter Andie. As a professional working to improve the lives of infants and families in the NICU where they must spend their first weeks (and often months), Kasey Mathews has made me painfully aware of how far we must still go to do better by the parents and their infants in our care. This book will make an important difference in spurring us on to realize the enormity of the experience of having a pre-term born infant."

—*Dr. Heidelise Als,*
Associate Professor at Harvard Medical School
and Director of Neurobehavioral Infant and Child Studies
at Children's Hospital Boston

"Kasey Mathews writes with unflinching honesty about the shock and shame of mothering a child born four months prematurely. Kasey brings readers in close as she careens between hospitals, a household, and a marriage, gradually discovering her willingness to try almost anything to help her baby survive. With humor, heart, and humanity, we witness a woman and her family who grow in dimension, capacity, and wisdom along with Andie's lungs, limbs, and life force. *Preemie* is a testament to what can happen when the rational mind cedes the notion of control and becomes open to alternatives...no matter how embarrassing they may once have seemed. Kasey Mathews' voice as a writer is as deep with feeling and complexity as is her family's story—both embracing the imperfect beauty, not of what happens to us, but what we choose to make of it. Through a series of small surrenders and forthright actions Kasey Mathews becomes the warrior you would want on your side."

—*Virginia Prescott, host of* Word of Mouth *public radio*
show and podcast

"After caring for many patients with their beloved children in the NICU, as well as suffering that same roller coaster ride with my own child, I can say that *Preemie* provides the most important thing: hope."

—*Fletcher Wilson, M.D., Chief of OB/GYN at Monadnock Community Hospital and Chairman of the Medical Advisory Board for Wide Horizons for Children*

"Kasey Mathews' authentic and boldly honest voice touched me deeply as a neonatal occupational therapist and mother. She taught me to never make assumptions about what our NICU parents are experiencing. *Preemie* unveils the silent trauma that comes with loving these fragile babies and the stunning joy that unfolds as they grow into strong (and often super-determined) children."

—*Sue Ludwig OTR/L, President and Founder of National Association of Neonatal Therapists*

Contents

◆

Part II

*To Lee, Tucker, and Andie, my traveling companions
on this wild and wondrous journey.*

◆

No snowflake ever lands in the wrong place.

Z E N P R O V E R B

✦

EVERYONE HAS A STORY. Mine began in November of 2000 when I thought I'd given birth to the smallest baby ever born. She arrived four months prematurely, weighing one pound, eleven ounces and measuring eleven inches long. Imagine a potato with tiny arms and legs. Several days after my daughter's birth, I mustered up the courage to ask a nurse if she'd ever seen a baby that little. When she replied, "Oh honey, this hospital floor is full of babies this small," I no longer felt quite so alone.

After my daughter was born, I longed for a compassionate woman who had been in my shoes to sit on the end of my hospital bed and share her story with me. It wouldn't matter how different or similar our stories were, just to have someone who understood what it was like to have a pregnancy end halfway through, resulting in a baby that didn't resemble any baby I'd ever seen. I wanted to see her nod in understanding as we discussed the daunting task of raising, loving, and believing in a child born at 25 weeks.

That woman never arrived. Due to hospital privacy rights, we were discouraged from even glancing at other babies or parents in the Neonatal Intensive Care Unit (or NICU). I was lost, incredibly lonely, and terribly wrought with guilt and fear.

So I'd like to sit on the end of your bed and share my story with you. Your story and mine are sure to be different, but if hearing my story allows you a moment away from yours, if it leaves you with a sense of hope, then this story was worth writing down.

✦

Part I

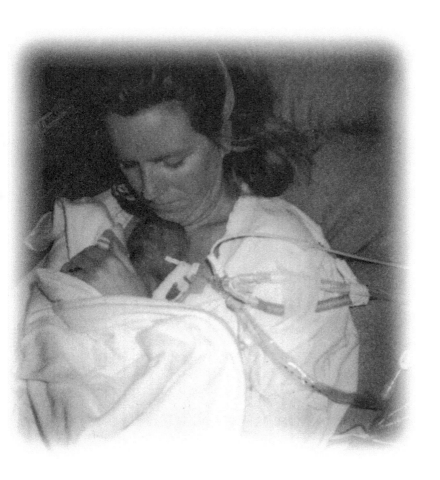

I

Hospital

✦

T HE CAR STOPPED in front of the hospital's main
entrance. I stared out the window. The revolving door
stood motionless, waiting for a push. When I looked at Lee,
his mouth was smiling, but his eyes were not. I leaned into
him, and he rested his lips on my forehead. Tucker's tiny hik-
ing boots swung back and forth, banging against the back of
my seat. A uniformed man tapped his pen against the glass
and motioned for us to move. As I pushed the car door open,
I could barely move my arms. The man held my elbow, and I
turned back to gaze at the car. "Wave to Mommy," Lee said.
I watched the station wagon move off in search of a parking
space.

The admissions procedure was unusually prompt. I sat
in the empty waiting room, knowing that tomorrow all these
seats would be bursting with ripe-bellied women waiting for
their scheduled Monday morning appointments. My hand
stroked my recently popped middle. A startling pain in my
lower back reminded me why I was there. With no one at
the desk, I wondered how anyone behind the closed double
doors would know I was waiting.

My gaze fell on the coffee table in front of me. A beautiful, bright-eyed baby smiled at me from the glossy cover

of a parenting magazine. I imagined her name—something with Rose in the middle, maybe Hannah Rose or Ashley Rose, or perhaps Mackenzie Rose. We stared at each other. She seemed to want to say something. Her pouty lips and arched eyebrows appeared concerned. Still rubbing my belly, I whispered down to her, "Is my baby okay?"

Her brilliant blue eyes continued to stare silently at me, and I suddenly knew my baby was *not* okay. I let out a quiet sound, somewhere between a gasp and a sob, and then a nurse called my name.

A young Asian doctor held her clipboard close and dutifully recorded my answers about previous pregnancies.

"One," I answered. "Born on his due date at eight pounds."

She leaned against the counter and scribbled. Her shiny hair fell like a black cape over her shoulders.

I explained the few instances of bleeding I'd had earlier in the pregnancy. She nodded but didn't write these down.

"Where is your pain on a scale of 1–10?" she asked.

"Three."

"Good." Her pen made a scratching noise across the paper. I had a sudden desire to knock the clipboard out of her hands. "Well your pain doesn't seem that bad," she said, dropping the clipboard on the counter and pushing up her sleeves. "I'll just do an exam before you go."

She'd just begun the exam when Lee walked in with two-year-old Tucker in his arms. My hospital gown was pulled up to my stomach and the doctor's head was between my legs. I smiled at them. Lee leaned back against the wall and offered me a wink. I was about to introduce him to the doctor, when

4

she let out a gasp. "Oh my God," she said, "you're three centimeters dilated."

I'm not sure who called them, but a bunch of nurses were suddenly in the room, scrambling around me. "What does this mean?" I asked. The nurse next to me was tearing apart the Velcro of a blood pressure cuff. "It means you're not going home until this baby is born."

"But it's November," I told her. "My baby isn't due until March." It was like I had a lead weight on my chest. I couldn't get a full breath. "I can't stay here until March." The nurse's hair was in tight curls that looked like rollers. "We've just got to stop this labor," she said patting my shoulder.

They lifted me from the exam table onto a gurney. Two nurses raised my legs into the air and held them there. I saw a large needle coming toward my back end and felt a sting and something cool spreading under my skin.

The nurse put the needle in a red container marked "CONTAMINATED." Lee shifted Tucker to his other arm. "A steroid," she said. "To help develop the baby's lungs."

The hot prick of an IV went into my right arm. Tucker started screaming. But when I reached for him, the nurse set my arm back on the bed. Her hand was cold. "Dad's got him," she said. Lee squeezed Tucker closer. "It's gonna be alright, babe," he said, backing out of the room, keeping his eyes on mine. "It's gonna be alright."

Still holding my legs in the air, several nurses took hold of the metal bars and wheeled me out the door, past Lee and Tucker, down the tight hallway. I heard Tucker's shrill voice, "What's happening, Daddy? What's happening to Mommy?"

When I tried to sit up, the nurse on my right pushed me down and kept her hand firmly on my chest.

"I can't stay here." I lifted my head. "I can't stay here until March." I pictured myself lying in a hospital bed for the next four months, stacks of discarded magazines at my side, a wall-mounted television airing nothing but soaps, and Tucker at home, dressed in his Spiderman pajamas, carrying his snuggly blue blanket from room to room, looking for his mama.

The bed was moving fast. "Who will take care of Tucker?" My question echoed off of the hallway walls.

"He'll be okay," a nurse answered.

The hallway grew dark like a cave. Dim overhead lights cast strange shadows across the nurses' faces.

"Why is this happening?" I asked. "What did I do?" My voice sounded far away.

"You didn't do anything." The nurse on my right held my hand without looking at me. "This isn't your fault." Their shoes squeaked as they jogged alongside me.

"I know I did something." The nurses exchanged a look. My body started shaking. I was so cold. "I never should have played paddle tennis."

"It's nothing you did," several nurses said at once.

I thought if I could figure out why this was happening, I could make it stop. I searched for clues, chronicling the past week's activities and ingestions. The bath I took Saturday must have been too hot. I ate sushi. Just vegetables, but maybe it was the ginger. "I put ginger on some sushi." They gripped my ankles tighter. I could see their hands on my legs, but realized I couldn't feel them.

Finally, I clutched a nurse's arm. She was walking backwards, facing me, guiding the gurney down the hall. I dug my fingers into her flesh. I needed to know she was real. She looked at me. Her eyes, framed in dark circles, softened. I thought I'd found my sympathetic audience. "You don't understand," I said to her in a more coherent, controlled voice. "This sort of thing doesn't happen to me."

She held my gaze for a moment, and I waited. A gold cross swung at the base of her neck.

She continued to look at me. And then she said, "It does now."

2

Beginnings

✦

"**I** HAVE A CRUSH ON LEE," my college roommate announced.

She sat on the floor painting her toenails baby-doll pink. I was on the bed, re-reading a back issue of *Rolling Stone*. "You know him, tall, cute, on the ski team." She dabbed polish on her baby toe. "Check him out and tell me what you think." She'd have a new crush next week, but I agreed anyway.

A week later, he was pouring beer at a party off campus, and I walked up to him. "Are you Lee?" I asked. He looked up and blinked. Right away, I noticed those long dark lashes and strong jawbone. *Mmmm*, I thought. "Yeah," he said, handing me a red plastic cup overflowing with white foam. "Okay," I said, then took the beer and walked away.

We wouldn't meet again until after graduation. I was teaching kindergarten in Boston and had gone to Colorado to ski with friends during my spring break. My cousin, Pete, came down from Jackson Hole and brought along a fellow ski instructor, Lee.

Pete announced that he and Lee planned to take on the mountains by day and the bars by night. But every day Lee skied at my side and at night, instead of shooting pool with Pete and the guys, he danced with us girls at cheesy disco bars.

Lee and I stayed up into the early morning hours, holding hands and whispering to each other. "Do you remember walking up to me at a party?" he asked. "Yes," I said, tracing my finger over the scar on his eyebrow. "You walked away and never even told me your name." He ran his thumb down the center of my nose and stopped on my lips. "I spent the next two years keeping my eye out for you. You've been hard to find."

When ski season ended, Lee drove his white VW Rabbit to Boston. We were inseparable, riding around on fat-tired mountain bikes, dancing in our living room to Joe Cocker's "Feeling Alright" and bar hopping through Harvard Square.

We rented a small red cottage in the woods west of Boston. I was teaching second grade and Lee was working at a bank downtown. We played house; hanging up curtains, stripping old furniture we found at the dump, and planting bulbs around the yard.

One Sunday in late fall a realtor led us into an empty farmhouse with a sign over the door that read "CIRCA 1802." The place had crooked door frames, cracked ceilings, and horsehair plaster walls. "Now this is a house I can sink my teeth into," Lee said, running his hand over the fireplace mantel. Within a week we'd signed a purchase offer and started learning about plumb lines, joint compound, and knob and tube wiring. We spent our evenings sanding, plastering, and painting, only taking off our dust masks for occasional kisses and sips of Corona.

One particularly late night, while paint fumes still danced in the air, I took off my mask. "We own a house, three cars, a dog, and a cat," I said. Lee held his paintbrush in mid-air while drips fell onto the plastic drop cloth below his feet. "Any time you want to ask me to marry you, I *will* say yes."

✦

For Lee's 28th birthday, I took him to dinner at our favorite hangout, J.C. Hilary's. I was rattling on about the weekly adventures in my classroom when he excused himself to the bathroom. While he was gone, I munched on my salad drenched in poppy seed dressing. He returned looking pale. "Okay." He gripped the table. "Kasey..."

"Yeah?" I asked, with my mouth full.

"Will you marry me?"

I'd waited seven years for him to say those words and at that moment I had a black poppy seed stuck between every tooth. "Ask me later," I mumbled hardly moving my lips.

"What?" he asked.

I covered my mouth with my hand and mumbled louder, "Ask me later."

"Okay." He sat down and started cutting his steak. "So what do you want to talk about now?"

We laughed so hard the waiter came over to see if everything was alright.

Later, we stood on a frozen pond in the woods near our home under a nearly full moon. I shook with cold and excitement. Lee wrapped me tightly in his arms and screamed out, "Kasey Mathews, I love you. Will you marry me?"

That time, I said yes.

At our June wedding, my bridesmaids wore short blue-

and-white polka-dotted dresses that swirled when they walked, and Kodiak, our fuzzy brown dog, ambled down the aisle with our rings tied to his collar. At the reception, I did cartwheels across the country club lawn in my puffy white dress, while Lee laughed and cheered in delight.

✦

Not much changed once we were married, except, being good, firstborn children, we began talking about the next logical step: a baby.

The pregnancy books told us to have sex every other day from the twelfth day to the sixteenth. Lee thought he had a better idea. If a little sex was good, a lot was sure to be better.

For six months we had sex on the eighth day of my cycle right on through to the sixteenth. During a college semester abroad in Africa, I'd studied predator behavior on the grassland plains. Typically, the male lion mounted the female, remained in that position for two to three days, and ejaculated over 500 times. It is said in Swahili, "Pole sana, simba," or "So sorry, lioness." In this case, I was the lioness, and by the sixth month, I couldn't stand the sight of Lee. If we were in the same room I'd sneer, "Don't touch me, don't even look at me."

But all this sex and no pregnancy didn't seem to bother Lee at all. In fact, he was rather chipper. One Sunday, he was out on the patio flipping burgers when I overheard him say to a friend, "Well, the longer it takes to get pregnant, the more you get to practice."

I scheduled an appointment with our Ob/Gyn the next day.

Dr. Shah, my dear, soft-spoken Indian doctor, met us later that week at the close of the day. He invited us into his small office. Lee sat in a corner chair, under the diagram of a vulva, crossing and uncrossing his legs. I sat next to him and put my hand on his knee. "You okay?" I whispered.

"Oh yeah, I'm great," he whispered back. "Couldn't be better. I love sitting in the office of my wife's vagina doctor."

Dr. Shah straightened some papers on his desk and pushed his glasses up. His hair was neatly parted on the side and combed down like a young boy's. "So," he began. "You're having trouble conceiving, is it?"

"We've been trying for six months," I said.

Pulling a paper out of the pile, Dr. Shah said, "Well, the blood tests show all your hormonal levels are normal."

"Could you repeat that again, and say it *louder* this time?" Lee asked.

Dr. Shah was confused.

"Kasey's convinced something's wrong with her," Lee said. "So if you wouldn't mind, please just repeat what you said."

In a louder, but still soft-spoken voice, Dr. Shah said again, "I've checked all your hormone levels, and everything is normal."

Lee put his hand on my shoulder. "Did you hear that? You are fine. Everything is fine."

Dr. Shah cleared his throat. "Well, Lee, this does mean you will have to masturbate in a cup."

Lee sat up taller in his chair. "I can do that."

"Good. I am glad you can," Dr. Shah said.

I bit my bottom lip, trying not to laugh.

"Before you go, I'd like to ask just a few more questions," Dr. Shah said.

"Fire away," Lee said.

Dr. Shah looked at the paper in front of him. "How often do you have intercourse?" he asked. "Are you monitoring your daily temperature?" And on and on as he moved through the list of questions. Lee sat quietly while I answered each one. Then Dr. Shah asked, "Do you remain lying down after sexual intercourse?"

"Wait," Lee put his hand on his chest and said with wide eyes, "you're supposed to have sex lying down?"

I crossed my arms and slid down in my chair, but Dr. Shah laughed. He reached over to pat my knee. "These appointments are certainly different when he comes along," he said.

As we walked out of his office, Dr. Shah called after us, "Don't worry you two. I have a feeling things are going to happen very soon."

And they did. Lee never had to masturbate in a cup. I was pregnant the next month. It turned out I was ovulating every month on the eighteenth or nineteenth day of my cycle, just when I'd been locking Lee back in his lion cage.

3

Babies

◆

OUR BIRTHING CLASS met every Wednesday night for eight weeks. Since I knew almost nothing about caring for a newborn, and Lee knew even less, we were sure the teacher, in her long, gauzy skirts and Birkenstock sandals, would find us a lost cause. Giddy and nervous, we ended up with a case of the giggles in nearly every class.

During the seventh week, each couple was given an old-fashioned, mercury-filled thermometer. Holding up a doll, our instructor explained that we should gently spread the baby's bottom cheeks and coax the thermometer into the baby's anus, holding the end of the thermometer so as not to push it in too far. The class watched her demonstrate without picking up our dolls. Why bother trying on a doll with a hard plastic bum? But when we heard a loud tapping noise, all of us turned and stared in disbelief as a heavy-set guy at the end of the table tried to jam his thermometer into his wide-eyed doll. Totally unaware of his audience, he continued his pursuit . . . until the glass snapped. Silver termina-tor-like balls scattered across the table. Everyone scrambled for safety to various corners of the room. The guy's wife had her face buried in her hands. The man next to me whispered, "Now there's an example of Darwinism at work." I felt bet-ter about our chances.

On our way out, the teacher warned us that the next class would focus on caesarean births and birth complications.

◆

Lee had been out with clients all day and arrived just moments before class began. When he walked in, I let out a big breath and stopped checking my watch. He smiled and waved from the doorway. I waved back. As he crossed the room, I noticed his face was red. He looked sunburned. "Hey, babe," he said as he sat down. His eyes were bloodshot. When he tried to take my hand, I pulled it away, folding my arms on top of my belly. "Where have you been?"

"Out with clients," he said.

"Out with clients where?"

The rest of the class pretended not to listen, but the room was so quiet I knew they were tuning in to our little exchange.

"On Boston Harbor," he said, with less confidence.

"What were you doing?"

He mumbled something about chartering a boat. "Didn't I tell you?" he asked. All day I'd pictured Lee sitting around stuffy conference tables. Now, the scenery changed and I saw him aboard a massive sailboat, reclining in the sun with skinny, bikini-clad women passing around drinks.

"You have beer on your breath," I hissed. I was a pissed-off pregnant woman. My cheeks burned, and I couldn't get comfortable in my seat. The guy who'd broken the thermometer looked delighted to have the spotlight on someone else.

Finally, the teacher called us to attention. Before she

began the lesson on complicated birth scenarios she asked, "Who would like a turn with the sympathy belly?" Before the words left her mouth, my hand shot in the air. "Lee would," I said. The class smiled.

The "sympathy belly" was a 25-pound canvas replica of the pregnant female form, complete with swollen breasts and two five-pound metal balls that rest directly on the bladder. Sweet redemption came in the form of my husband standing in front of the entire class, looking very pregnant in a denim jumper.

Once the snickers subsided, our teacher pressed "Play" on the VCR and the screen began flashing unnerving images of doctors in green scrubs, hovering over terrified, birthing women. I should have paid attention. I should have felt uncomfortable. I should have felt scared by what I saw. But instead, the image of my ridiculous husband sporting a big, pregnant belly delighted me beyond measure. Besides, nothing like that would ever happen to us.

The class was silent as the video played on. Then Lee leaned over, his warm breath tickling my neck, and whispered, "I'm *dying* to play with these big boobies."

I exploded with laughter in the middle of a film about birth complications.

◆

Several months later, John Tucker arrived on his due date, weighing an even eight pounds. Before the umbilical cord was cut, the midwife placed him on my chest. He looked up at me with big, round eyes. My first thought was, *He's real.*

Lee was jumping up and down in the background, his hands raised in the air. I couldn't take my eyes off the baby staring back at me. "I'm your mommy," I whispered and his eyes seemed to say, "I know."

He was born on a Sunday morning in late summer. That afternoon, the Red Sox played down the road. From our room on the tenth floor, we ate French toast with maple syrup and watched the baseball game on the enormous screen that towered above Fenway Park.

"This place is like a hotel," my father said, snapping another picture of Tucker.

"Yeah," Lee nodded. "You want to grab me a beer from the mini-bar?"

My father took the camera from his eyes. "You gotta be shitting me," he said. "This place has a bar?"

We all laughed and basked in the joy of celebrating the arrival of a healthy baby.

I'd never really been a baby person. I wasn't a natural like everyone else seemed to be. I found motherhood both amazing and terrifying. Whenever someone asked if I wanted to hold their baby, I always thought, *Why?* and politely declined. So it surprised and startled me how enamored I was with my own little guy.

Still, it took some time to find my rhythm as a new mom. I watched myself trying to play the role as I thought it should be played. We'd get together with other moms who I thought all looked and acted like mothers should. Sitting within their circle, I felt like an imposter, and not a very good one at that. I studied their actions and analyzed mine in comparison, hoping to find that elusive *something* I thought was missing. They had their perfectly packed diaper bags filled with travel wipes, hand sanitizer, and sets of spare clothing. I was happy just to have remembered the baby.

I spent a good part of every day with Tucker in a jogger stroller, walking around town. At home, I put on Joni Mitchell and danced around the kitchen with him in my arms. We lay on a patchwork quilt in the backyard and studied the green grass growing beneath us. Our time together was unrushed and serene.

Yet, just as I was starting to feel comfortable in my new role, an alarm must have sounded, or a memo sent out, because suddenly everyone was talking about second babies. All my mom-friends were either pregnant or planning to be, while I was still just figuring out this whole first baby thing.

I guess Lee got the memo, because he started riding that second baby train, too. There was this now-or-never mentality, and like most baby stuff, it made little sense to me. Lee's argument was based on sibling age spans.

"Even if we got pregnant now, the kids would be two-and-a-half years apart," he said, bouncing Tucker on his knee. "Besides, it took so long to get pregnant with Tuck, who knows how long it could take? We should at least try."

I put my hands on my hips. "Oh, so you can practice again?"

Lee smiled.

For a reluctant, first-time mom still finding her way, the concept of a second baby seemed incredibly daunting. But I knew there was reason to Lee's logic. We might as well start trying sooner than later. On my daily walks, I imagined a calendar in my head. With at least six months to conceive, and nine months to grow, a baby was well over a year away. By then, Tuck would be close to three. He and I would still have lots of time together before anything changed.

So I agreed to start trying.

I was pregnant in the first month.

4

Home

✦

I WENT FOR MY FIRST DOCTOR'S APPOINTMENT
at eight weeks.

"Congratulations," Dr. Shah said. "And how is that husband of yours?" We laughed and I assured him his friend Lee
was doing just fine.

The appointment was routine. He confirmed the pregnancy and told me everything looked great. Dr. Shah's nurse
checked the calendar on the wall, "March 12th," she said
with a smile. "Spring is the perfect time for a new baby." I
smiled back, thinking how far off spring was.

After we'd adjusted to the surprising quickness of conception, we laid out our battle plan. We'd have an entire
summer, fall, and winter to renovate the upstairs of our
two-family house, converting the apartment living room
and kitchen into our master bedroom and bathroom. "If I
start in December," our contractor said, "I'll be out of there
by mid-February." We'd have a whole month left before the
baby arrived.

Two weeks after I saw Dr. Shah, I had some light bleeding. The same thing had happened early in my pregnancy with
Tuck, so I wasn't too concerned. But the bleeding persisted
for a few days, and Dr. Shah asked me to come in for an
ultrasound. When the black-and-white screen revealed the

tiny baby floating in my uterus, its miniscule heart rapidly beating away, Lee leaned over and kissed my cheek.

"There could be three reasons for the bleeding," Dr. Shah said, washing his hands in the little steel sink. "It could be the result of a miscarried twin." I saw rolled footage of the airport scenes my cousins and I endured throughout our childhoods: Mom and Aunt Mimi, sobbing in each other's arms, then letting go, only to run back to the familiar safety of the other twin's embrace before finally boarding the plane. I wondered if my baby would spend its life longing for that missing sibling.

"Or," Dr. Shah said, wiping his hands on a paper towel, "It might be a uterine hematoma, or bruise." I didn't think to ask how my uterus might have become bruised. He threw the paper towel in the trash and crossed his arms over his white lab coat. "Or," he said, "Perhaps the fetus attached, unattached, and reattached in a different place on the uterine wall." I pictured a fetus with tiny rock climbing equipment.

"Whatever the reason, we'll never know for sure." He patted my shoulder. "For now you should go home and stay off your feet." Lee and I looked over at Tucker straining to get out of his stroller. *Yeah right*, I thought.

I put my daily walks on hold and, within a few days, the bleeding slowed and soon stopped. When I was on my feet again, I turned my attention back to Tucker. I wanted to make the most of our time together. A friend had told me when you have one child you can sort of live your old pre-kid life. "Two kids," he'd said, "Forget it. You're in deep."

In early September, I was about 15 weeks along. We loaded up the Volvo wagon with towels, sand toys, and the portacrib. Our bikes stood at attention on the roof of the car as we headed to Cape Cod. I looked out at the water under the Sagamore Bridge. "I can't wait to take long bike rides by the beach," I said.

Shortly after we arrived, I parked the car under the apple trees in front of our rental house. It wasn't until I heard the horrible crunching sound that I remembered the bikes were on the roof rack. Sitting in the driver's seat with my head in my hands, I bawled while Lee assured me our vacation wasn't ruined. "Just our bikes," he said with a smile. As we stored the mangled bikes in the garage, I asked no one in particular, "Why did this have to happen?"

The next day I had my answer: I started bleeding again. I imagined my angels, rubbing their hands together as they plotted to keep me off my bike, *ah, the apple trees!*

The bleeding was heavier this time, and Dr. Shah no longer *suggested* I stay off my feet, he *insisted*. After five days of bed rest, both the bleeding and our vacation came to an end.

Back home, Tuck and I played in the fallen maple leaves. I picked out paint colors for the upstairs and Lee started the final semester of his MBA program. He'd been working his way through business school part-time for four years. Somehow, he'd managed to squeeze classes into his long workdays, two-hour commute, house renovations, and life with a little one. When we found out I was pregnant, he'd loaded up the fall semester with his two remaining classes. They were grueling. The new approach to MBA programs emphasized working on group projects, but two of the four members in his group weren't keeping up, so he was doing his work plus theirs.

By Thanksgiving we were ready for a break. We drove home to my parents' house in upstate New York where my brother, John, and his girlfriend, Lollie, were coming from Manhattan. There'd been an early snowfall, and we were all excited to sled and ski on the golf course behind my parents' house.

When we arrived at the big white house where I'd grown up, Mom and Dad's overweight yellow Lab ran out to greet us, circling our legs and whacking us with his tail.

"Kase, you're tiny," my mom said. She stood on her toes to kiss me. Her gold bangles sang as she reached out to touch my belly. "You're barely showing." I wondered if this was a good thing. Her friends always bragged how they'd gained only about 12 pounds during their pregnancies, and then added with a laugh that they'd smoked cigarettes and drank gin and tonics, too. I had no idea how much weight I'd gained. During my check-ups I stood backwards on the scale and told the nurse I didn't want to know. I just wanted to eat and enjoy myself.

"*Oof,*" Dad said, as he picked up Tuck. He was still limping on the knee we begged him to have replaced. Tucker grabbed at his glasses as my Dad sang "Old MacDonald" and carried him into the house. We lifted bags out of the car and followed them inside. Walking through the spotless white kitchen with the dog's bed plopped on the Oriental rug, I had that strange sense of not knowing which house was really home. The one Lee and I were creating in Massachusetts? Or this one with the shelves full of family photographs, the cozy den where my sister and I had watched *Love Boat* on Friday nights, and the basement game room where Dad and I played our ongoing ping-pong matches?

We spent the next two days preparing for turkey day, visiting old friends, sledding, and playing paddle tennis while everyone swooned over Tucker, the first grandchild. I'd really been looking forward to my favorite meal: a fat, roasted turkey with all the fixings. But on Thanksgiving Day, my clothes were too tight and I felt full and uncomfortable. "You okay, babe?" Lee asked when he noticed I'd barely nibbled at the food. "Yeah." I pushed my plate away. "I just feel kind of icky." I put my napkin on the table. "I think I'll go upstairs and lie down." When I stood up, my mom looked over. "Look," she said. "Your belly popped."

All week, we'd planned to cross-country ski, but the day after Thanksgiving, I couldn't muster the energy. I wasn't really sick, just feeling dull and queasy. I kept rubbing my newly rounded belly, trying to will myself back into my own skin. Instead of skiing, I tried a nap, a bath, and a ginger ale. Nothing made me feel better. Lying under a blanket on the king-sized bed in my parent's bedroom, I stared at the ceiling. My mom's friends had stopped to see Tucker, and I could hear their laughter coming from downstairs.

Lee came in to check on me. Sitting beside me on the bed, he pushed my hair back from my forehead, leaned over, and kissed it. "I want to go home," I told him. He nodded. "We'll leave tomorrow."

We left Saturday evening, hoping to avoid holiday traffic and get Tuck to sleep through most of the trip. Though I shifted positions constantly, my lower back was killing me and I couldn't get comfortable. Finally, I decided to drive. I was in too much pain to sleep.

"This feels like the labor I had with Tucker," I said to the dark car.

Lee woke up and rubbed his eyes. "Maybe we should call the doctor." (Later, Lee revealed he'd debated about driving us straight to an emergency room.)

"No." I didn't know if I was assuring him, or myself. "I think I'm just uncomfortable being in the car."

We got home after midnight and went straight to bed. I barely slept. Throughout the night, I drifted in and out of totally bizarre dreams.

I felt even worse in the morning and phoned my Ob/ Gyn's office. Because it was Sunday, the office was closed and the woman on the phone told me to go directly to Brigham and Women's Hospital in Boston, where the doctors were doing weekend rounds. This was where I'd delivered Tuck, almost an hour away. What I really wanted to do was climb back in bed and recuperate with some sleep. "How about I go in the morning?" I asked. But she insisted I go in right away.

Assuming we'd be in and out of the hospital on an early Sunday morning, I grabbed a diaper and a few snacks for Tuck. I didn't want to leave home. Nervous and shaky, I stood at the back door watching Lee get Tuck in the car. Lee looked up at me. "Come on, babe," he said, and I hesitantly stepped forward.

5

Birth

✦

O N   T H A T   D R E A R Y   N O V E M B E R   D A Y   when Lee took
me to the hospital, I went from a blissfully naive, ex-
pectant mother halfway through her pregnancy to a woman
whose pregnancy could end at any moment. I knew nothing
about premature labor. I knew babies could be born early,
but I didn't know they could be born 15 *weeks* early. I had no
idea what a preemie looked like. I hadn't read the pregnancy
books. I'd eaten healthy food, slept well, exercised, and created a calm, comfortable environment that I thought would
protect the growing baby inside me. It had worked with
Tucker, so I was sure it would work with baby number two.

After the nurse told me that yes, in fact, things like this
do happen to me, I stayed silent. The nurses looked straight
ahead as they pushed my bed. We took a right off the hallway
into a room with shadowy yellow walls. The building outside
the window was so close that I could see the desks and filing
cabinets in the dark offices. While doctors and nurses came
in and out of the room, attaching me to tubes and wires, Lee
set the broken remote control on the bedside table and stood
in front of the TV with Tucker in his arms, reaching up to
change the channels. I kept staring at the clock. It looked like

the one I'd had in my classroom, mounted high on the wall with a black second hand clicking past the numbers. Lee's parents and mine were stuck in an ice storm in upstate New York, the same storm that would have stranded us somewhere along the New York State Thruway if we hadn't left the night before. Only a few stations came in, and Lee finally settled on a show about dog training. He put Tuck in a chair next to me, hoping it would hold his attention.

The admitting doctor examined me again and began talking about a caesarean section, while a labor and delivery nurse moved quietly around the room, busying herself with monitors and machinery. The moment the doctor walked out, the nurse turned to us. "You did not hear this from me," she said, pushing her brown bangs from her eyes and glancing at the door. "But I've been at this hospital for over 20 years, and that doctor has only been here six months. She's good, but she's young. Every moment you keep that baby inside you is vital. Don't let them take that baby out unless they absolutely have to."

Lee and I nodded obediently. Tucker turned away from the TV and studied her with his wide, hazel eyes.

"And hope for a girl," she said, checking the IV bag. "They have stronger lungs." She wrote something on a chart and walked out the door, as though the conversation never happened.

A girl. I knew I wasn't having a girl. Years before, when Lee and I were visiting Santa Fe, New Mexico, and the idea of a baby was just a conversation between us, I had a dream so real that I felt sure it was a premonition. I was walking through the market in Santa Fe's old town and wandered into a crowded party in a small, adobe house. I didn't know anyone there, but an old woman, dressed in native clothes with colorful beading, walked straight out of a plaster wall to me. "You will have two boys," she said before disappearing back into the wall. I'd woken to a turquoise New Mexico morning and told Lee about the dream. A girl was out of the question.

Our delivery nurse set a glass of water by my bedside. "A team from pediatrics is coming," she said in her quick voice. "What they say will scare the shit out of you." She didn't have any makeup on, and for some reason this comforted me. "Stay positive and remember," she put the call button within arm's reach, "you're in Boston. If you have to deliver a preemie, you're in one of the best hospitals in the world. Statistics are nationwide, and the stats in Boston are much better."

I looked at Lee, who nodded. "Okay," he said. "Thank you."

Walking out, the nurse almost bumped into my friend Karen, who came through the door with her son, Matthew, trailing behind her. Tucker jumped up and ran toward them. She winked at me and squatted down to ruffle Tuck's hair. I tried to smile back, but it was a thin, sorry excuse for a smile. I saw myself through Karen's eyes: a woman in a flimsy hospital gown, hooked up to wires and monitors. She knew where I was headed. I was on my way to that exclusive club whose members knew suffering, loss, and grief. Karen was a member. "Tuck, you're coming home with us tonight," she was saying. Her layered chestnut hair framed her soft, freckled face. "Okay, buddy?" Tucker nodded eagerly and grabbed at Matthew's Red Sox hat.

Karen stood up and wrapped her arms around Lee. I remembered how I sought her out in our new mom's group because of her big, signature smile. She was delighted at being a new mom, and I was drawn to her light, wanting to know the secret of her happiness. Matthew was just 10 weeks older than Tucker, and we talked about our lives before kids, our careers, and our husbands. I'd been intrigued when she told me she was 15 years younger than her husband. "How'd you guys meet?" I pictured them on a museum tour or in a painting class.

"A bereavement group," she'd said.

She'd been married six months when her first husband's heart stopped beating and refused to start again. She was twenty-nine. Two years later, she met Pete, a widower with four teenage kids. After a year of dinners and movies, they were married on a small Caribbean island. Baby Matthew arrived a year later.

I watched her break away from Lee. She walked over and stood at the end of my bed.

"Oh, Kase," she said, and touched my foot. "How ya doing?"

"I'm okay," I said.

She gently rubbed my ankle while Lee explained where she'd find Tucker's pajamas and toothbrush.

"How are you like this?" I'd asked her that day.

She'd been sitting calmly with Matthew curled on her

lap, and her smile had faded just a bit. "It's taken me a long time to get here," she'd said.

Watching Karen from the bed of that labor and delivery room on the third floor of a hospital in the middle of a busy, bustling city, I thought about what she had been through, and realized that things like this really did happen to people like me. I watched Lee pick up Tuck. "You ready to go, big guy?" Karen smiled at him and Tucker looked over at me. "Come give me a hug," I told him. I had to push away tubes and wires in order for him to get up on the bed with me. I rubbed the soft fleece of his coat and smelled his hair. "Be good, sweet man." I kissed his head. And then he was through my hands and heading to the door, gripping Karen's finger in his.

✦

In their matching white coats, the three pediatric doctors looked like clones of one another. They walked in with stethoscopes around their necks, carrying clipboards, with their hair too neat and their shoes making squeaking sounds on the linoleum. Standing in a semicircle around my bed, they began spewing statistics. I saw their mouths moving, but refused to listen, imagining them whispering about brain bleeds, cerebral palsy, wheelchairs, and ten-year-olds in diapers. *These aren't doctors*, I thought to myself. *They're freakin' medical mathematicians—all numbers, calculations, and statistics.*

Do over, I wanted to scream. *Why are we doing this?* I wanted ed to ask. *Why can't we just move on and have another baby?* But I'd never say those words aloud, even to Lee. And I wondered what sort of mother would ever think those thoughts.

Before the doctors left, one of them tapped the metal bed rail with his wedding ring. "Thirty weeks," he said. His ring sounding like a warning bell. "Just try and get to 30 weeks." He pushed his glasses further up on his nose. I could see the raw red mark where he must have done that over and over. "All the baby's major organs will be fully developed at 30 weeks," he said. For the first time since they'd entered the room, I nodded. I could do that. It was a plan, a goal, something to strive for.

Throughout the day, the young admitting doctor continued to check my progress and we repeatedly refused the caesarean option every time she brought it up. I was sick and swollen from being pumped full of magnesium sulfate to slow the labor, and my mouth had a metallic taste. The labor pains kept coming.

I could barely feel Lee's hand through my puffy fingers. Laying my head back on the pillow, I said, "We'd better start talking about names." Lee shook his head. "You're going to get to thirty weeks," he told me. I looked at the monitor strapped to my belly and followed the cord to the bright red digital numbers flashing on the screen. I wondered what they all meant. "Let's pick a couple out," I said. "Just in case."

During my first pregnancy, from the moment of conception we'd talked about names. It drove Lee crazy that I wanted to have one picked out so long before I got to the hospital, but I kept picturing an impatient nurse, tapping her foot and chomping her gum, pencil and pad in hand, waiting to take my order. I'd panic from the pressure and blurt out, "I'll have a cheeseburger," when I really wanted a Caesar salad. It was a week before Tucker was due when I grew tired of the names we'd picked out and wanted to start over. Lee vowed during our second pregnancy we wouldn't discuss names until the last month. *Oops.*

He sat down on the edge of the bed and picked up my hand. "This baby will need a strong name."

I remembered the journal I'd kept sitting on my bookshelf in our bedroom during my first pregnancy. On the second page I'd carefully drawn a line down the center, writing "GIRL" across the right side and "BOY" across the left. I went through the list of unused girl names. Lee shrugged. I twisted his wedding band around on his finger. "What about Andie?"

"Andie." He looked out the window at the overcast November day. "It sounds strong. But she needs a more . . ." He squinted, like he always did when he was trying to think hard, "Proper first name."

"We could use Anne, your Mom's middle name, with a middle name that starts with D. Anne D.—Andie."

"Maybe." He didn't sound convinced.

I reached up and ran a finger along his jaw line. "What about Daniel?" Lee's childhood friend Daniel who'd died right after college. He shook his head.

"Babe, this baby's gonna need all the angels he or she can get." I let my fingers rest on his cheek. His eyes trailed back to mine. He looked at me for a long time before nodding slowly, and we agreed without really agreeing, because we thought we'd have more time. We never did decide on a boy's name.

Throughout the day, Lee sat by my bed, phoning his parents, my parents, my brother, his brother, my sister, and our neighbors and friends. I stared at the TV, trying to tune out his end of the conversations. "She's hanging in there . . . trying to stop the labor . . . doctors say 30 weeks." A nurse delivered a sandwich that Lee picked at while we stared at a basketball game. "Maybe I should call Fletch," he said pushing the plate away.

Fletch was a college friend who'd surprised us by going to medical school. Now he was an Ob/Gyn resident in Rochester, New York. I had known his wife, Holly, since childhood. She and Lee had been on our college ski team together. Holly and Fletch knew firsthand what we were going through. Their first baby, Ford, died five weeks after birth, just a few months after Tucker was born. Holly was due with their second baby in a week.

"No way, Lee. You can't."

He pushed his hair off his forehead. "They'd want to know, Kase."

I let out a big breath and watched him pick up the phone. There was the regular small talk and then he said, "Hey listen, I don't want to bother you guys, but I thought you should know . . ." I listened as he explained that he wanted them to feel included but not burdened. Then he told them the situation. He was silent for a long time, twisting the phone cord around his fingers. When he got off the phone, he rubbed his hand over his eyes. "What'd he say?" I asked. Lee turned to me. "He said he wants to be included every inch of the way." I nodded. "And he said what the delivery nurse said." He picked my hand up. "Keep that baby inside and shoot for 30 weeks." I couldn't talk. Lee brought my hand to his lips and kissed each knuckle. "We're gonna be alright," he told me.

Years later, Holly would confess that Fletcher had hung up the phone and touched her swollen belly. "We might be going to a funeral," he'd said.

By late afternoon, we'd put off the admitting doctor's urgent requests to perform a c-section three times. At 5:45 she stood just inside the doorway and reported that she was due to end her shift. I stole a glance at Lee and saw relief cross his face. She pulled her clipboard to her chest. "Well . . . she said. "Good luck." As she turned to leave, she looked back. "The doctor coming on for the night shift is Dr. Shah." I sat up in bed. "My Dr. Shah?" I asked.

When he stepped through the doorway, his warm eyes surveyed me from behind those metal-framed glasses. The lights in the room seemed to soften and the bed beneath me felt more forgiving as my body relaxed into it. When I whispered his name, it came out with a mixture of hope and despair.

He walked over to my bedside. "Hullo, Kate," he said quietly. He always called me by my given name. Whenever a teacher or doctor read my given name off a paper, I quickly corrected them, but Dr. Shah's accent made it sound musical and light.

"Hullo, Lee," he said. Lee reached over from the other side of my bed and they shook hands over my belly.

Dr. Shah placed his hand on my shoulder, the warmth of

it spreading into my tight muscles. I wanted him to tell me everything was going to be alright, but his smile was cheerless and his brow furrowed. He looked to Lee and back to me. "Ah, Kate, if anyone can do this," he said, "It is sure to be you." I felt a surge of confidence rise up from the lower recess of my back. I could do this. I looked at Lee on my left and Dr. Shah on my right and thought, *I'll show these men in my life just how strong I am.*

"Forget 30 weeks," I said. "I'm going to take this baby all the way to 40."

When Dr. Shah left to check on other patients, Lee took my hand again. "I know you can do this, babe."

Dr. Shah returned repeatedly throughout the night. Every time he checked the monitors, my contractions had spread out and lessened in intensity. At first they were six minutes apart, then seven. Reverse labor is a full-term mother's worst nightmare, but what I was hoping for against all odds. Around midnight, when Dr. Shah came in to check my progress, I asked if he had any memory of a boy or girl from our ultrasounds. He shook his head.

Finally, I fell asleep. The next time I woke, Dr. Shah was walking in and the light from the hallway shone on the clock. It was just after three in the morning. Lee had fallen asleep in the chair next to me, and he stirred in his sleep. Dr. Shah walked over to the glowing monitors. "Hi," I whispered. "Sorry to wake you," he said, patting my arm. "I'll just check your progress and let you get back to sleep." I watched him read the monitors and waited. "Eight minutes." He looked down at me. "You're doing it, Kate."

At 6:30 in the morning a nurse came in to check my blood pressure. Lee stood by my bedside, sipping coffee from a Styrofoam cup. The nurse looked up at the clock on the wall. "It's coming up on 24 hours that you've held off labor." She smiled. And then, at that exact moment, I felt a warm gush of water between my legs.

My water broke.

The nurse ran out of the room. Lee looked confused. Within seconds, doctors and nurses flooded the room, pushing him out of the way. "The baby's heartbeat is dropping," Dr. Shah said. "We've got to get that baby out."

A nurse tugged at my gown until it was above my swollen stomach. I felt her squirt a glob of cold gel just above my pubic line. She held a razor in her hand and as she drew her first, quick stroke, I heard myself say, "Oh, I really prefer to wax." The nurse looked up at me with shocked eyes. Apparently not the time for sarcasm. I felt myself leave my body. I wasn't there. That wasn't me. There wasn't really a baby. This was a play. A made-for-TV drama with me in the starring role. Any moment, a director would call out "cut," and we'd break for coffee and doughnuts.

Minutes later, I was on a metal table in an operating room, surrounded by nurses and doctors. I counted six nurses and six doctors, some pediatric, some labor and delivery. Dr. Shah was there, which made me feel somewhat calmer, or maybe it was the cocktail of drugs coursing through my veins. He was standing at my belly with a scalpel in his hand when I asked him where Lee was. "Oh my goodness," he said. "We forgot the husband."

Lee had been told to stand in the hallway. In the chaos, they'd forgotten him. The double doors to the OR swung open and he was at my side, looking drawn and pale in a pair of faded green scrubs and a paper shower cap. "I'm proud of you," he said, looking into my eyes. I looked back at him. *Don't you see I failed?* I asked him silently. *I'm about to give birth, four months before I'm supposed to. Why would you ever be proud of me?* When I didn't respond, he said it again. "I'm proud of you."

"Remember, you won't hear the baby cry," a doctor from pediatrics called out. He stood behind Dr. Shah with two other doctors. I couldn't see his eyes, only the reflection of the lights in his glasses, "We'll have to intubate immediately."

"Intubate?" I looked up at Lee.

"It's okay," he squeezed my hand. "They have to put a breathing tube in the baby's lungs."

"Do you know what you're having?" the nurse on my left asked.

Lee and I shook our heads.

A large gray curtain in the shape of a fan was placed over my belly, dividing my upper half from my lower. Dr. Shah looked over the curtain and said something about a uterine cut, one way as opposed to the other, due to the baby's size. I didn't know what he was talking about, and with the drugs swirling through me I didn't care, but Lee left my side and went to stand behind the curtain with Dr. Shah.

The room was quiet except for the nurse beside me. She patted my arm and asked, "You doing okay?"

My eyes were squeezed shut. I wished she'd be quiet. I

imagined I was home with Tucker, lying in our bed listening to him say, "Hi baby" to my belly. *This can't be happening,* I kept thinking. I was so cold that my teeth chattered and, even with my eyes closed, the lights penetrated the skin of my lids.

"The baby's out," Dr. Shah said. I opened my eyes and saw the pediatricians turn away from me and move to the counter behind them. I assumed they had the baby. The room was nearly silent. Then we heard a cry. A quick, high-pitched cry like the lid of a box had opened and quickly shut. Lee looked over the curtain. *It's a sign,* I told him with my eyes. *A sign that our baby is strong.* He nodded.

After the cry, the room stayed quiet. The pediatric doctors lined up at the counter doing whatever it was they had to do with our baby. Nurses bustled about the room. The nurse on my left never left my side. "You doin' okay?" she asked again. I turned to look at her and saw for the first time how watery her eyes were. "No," I said. "I'm not." My light blue hospital gown had slid down my arm and she smoothed it back up on my shoulder. She never asked me again how I was doing. "Do you know if it was a boy or girl?" I asked. She frowned and shook her head. "Lee," I called out, suddenly desperate to know. "Was it a boy or a girl?"

When he looked over the curtain, his eyebrows shot up like he'd just remembered I had an upper half. He whispered to Dr. Shah, who shrugged his shoulders and said, "They took the baby so fast I didn't have time to look." The question rippled around the operating room. "A girl," one of the pediatric doctors finally called out without turning from the counter. "You have a baby girl."

Words that often lend themselves to champagne and cigars were met instead with the depressed smiles of several OR nurses who turned to look my way. The nurse securing my IV asked if we had a name.

Lee came over and stood by my shoulder. We both knew a name made this baby real. I moved my mouth but couldn't speak. I wasn't sure if we'd really agreed on a name. Lee picked up my hand, and I watched as first his eyes, then his whole face, took on an expression of certainty. In a proud voice, he announced, "Her name is Anne. Anne Daniel, and we'll call her Andie."

The nurse on my left patted my arm, "That's pretty," she said. Dr. Shah looked over the curtain. "It's a good name."

"We're going to move the baby up to the NICU," the doctor with the glasses said. The team of pediatric doctors and several nurses moved quickly toward the OR doors. I assumed they had our baby with them, but I never saw her. The double doors pushed open and the team moved through to the other side. The doors swung shut and our baby was gone.

6

Trains

◆

AT FOUR YEARS OLD I was attacked by an Afghan
hound. It happened after my Aunt Harriet's wedding
reception. I was a flower girl, dressed in soft blue cotton,
my blond hair hanging down my back. A framed picture of
my Dad and me at the wedding rests on a bookshelf in my
parents' den. My father looked like Rock Hudson in his tux,
holding my hand, leading me to the dance floor.

After the reception, we went back to Nam and Gramp's
house on Farmer Street. Mom put me in pajamas and then to
bed, but hearing my cousins playing with the neighborhood
kids, I snuck out to join them.

When my parents heard the screams and saw the bloody,
fair-haired child cradled in Uncle Glenn's arms, they thought
my cousin Peter was hurt. I only remember bright lights,
scary green masked men, and heavy swinging doors that
kept my parents on the other side.

They sewed 49 stitches in the left side of my face—two
sets below my eye, another by my ear, two sets beside my
mouth, and the last one on my neck, along my jugular vein.
Apparently when the dog attacked, I'd fallen face forward on
the driveway. Mom always said, if I'd landed face up I would
have been killed. Dad said the three days and nights I slept

between them, whimpering in pain, were the longest of his life.

I still had the stitches in my face when Dad and I went out one day to the P&C for groceries. I ran over to hug a dog tied to a signpost, but before I could pet him, Dad grabbed me by the arm and yanked me away. Squatting down, he put his big hands on my shoulders and looked me in the eye. "If you *ever* do that again," he shook his finger at me until I thought I'd cry. "I'll pull your pants down and spank you right here."

When I had Tucker, I finally understood why my father scolded me that way, why he often touched my barely visible scars and offered to pay for collagen injections and other plastic-surgery procedures.

As I lay staring at the ceiling in the recovery room just after Andie was born, I remembered my father's face that day at the grocery store, and I remembered years later watching a friend hold her newborn and tell me she would stand in front of a moving train to protect him. I didn't have kids yet and wondered if she'd lost her mind. Now I knew I'd stand in front of 10 moving trains and a thousand Afghan hounds to protect Tucker, but this half-done baby I'd never even seen? I tried counting the dots in the acoustical tile to stop these thoughts, but couldn't make it past seven before my eyes blurred with tears.

Lee hung up the phone. "Elizabeth and Todd are on their way."

"No," I wiped my palm across my cheeks. "Please, call them back and tell them not to come. I don't want them to see me."

Lee squatted beside my bed and brushed the hair from my face. "They drove all night through this storm," he said quietly. "I'm not going to tell them to turn back. Besides, they're only a few minutes away and they want to be here with us."

When Lee's brother and his wife walked in, I tried to sit up and smile. Lee and Todd held each other for a long time. Elizabeth squeezed my hand. "How are you doing?" she asked, setting a tray of Starbucks down on the table next to me. "Well," I started, but didn't finish. She handed Lee a coffee. The bitter smell lodged in the back of my throat and made it hard for me to swallow.

They stood around me, drinking their coffee. Elizabeth moved behind the bed to rub my shoulders. I stiffened. I didn't want her to touch me. I didn't deserve her kindness. Something I had or had not done caused my baby to come early, and I deserved to be punished, not comforted. My body had failed me and everyone else. But when her hands reached my neck they were so soft, I couldn't resist the tenderness. I let myself close my eyes and relax for just a little bit.

We all turned when a nurse appeared in the doorway. "Ready to see your baby?" she asked cheerfully.

"No," I said.

The room went still. All eyes turned to me.

"Oh," the nurse pushed up her funky reading glasses. "Are you sure?" she had a perky voice that sounded sing-songy in the sterile room. "Because it's really important for Mom and baby to see each other."

"No, thanks. I'm okay," I said, as if she were passing a tray of hors d'oeuvres.

I don't know why she bothered asking. She looked from Elizabeth to Lee and finally to his brother, and then she marched into the room and the four of them began to move my bed.

"I said I don't want to go."

No one answered.

When I started to protest again, the nurse kicked the brake off the bed. "Well, let's just get you started and see if you change your mind."

Lee and Todd pushed the bed from behind while the nurse led the way. Elizabeth walked beside me, holding my hand. The bed navigated the narrow corridors past swirling signs and faces, causing my head to spin. I felt like I was rocking in the hull of a boat. I thought of the poem my second grade students memorized every year. I silently recited it in my head. "My Bed is a Boat," they would begin. "by Robert Louis Stevenson."

> My bed is like a little boat;
> Nurse helps me in when I embark;
> She girds me in my sailor's coat
> And starts me in the dark.

> At night, I go on board and say
> Good night to all my friends on shore;
> I shut my eyes and sail away
> And see and hear no more.

My bed and its band of followers came to a stop in front of a set of double doors labeled "NICU." At the time, those letters meant nothing to me, but once I was pushed through those doors, they came to mean everything.

My bed moved down a hallway, through another set of doors, and into a brightly lit room filled with machines and medical staff. They stopped my bed in front of a plastic box. Another nurse was waiting. Like a model on a game show, she greeted me with a smile. *Show her what she's won, Johnnie.* She opened the box. "There's your baby," chirped the transport nurse.

Splotches flashed in my vision and my eyes went blurry. What was inside that box was something out of a sci-fi movie. I imagined a mad scientist, surrounded by boiling pots and smoking glass beakers, making these babies in the adjoining room. That couldn't be a human baby, so pale, translucent, and alien-like. That could not be *my* baby. And just as I had this thought, I threw up all over myself. Other people in the room turned our way. The perky nurse went silent. And then she quickly wheeled my bed back out of the NICU.

Throughout the rest of the day, the mixture of drugs and the vision of my daughter swirled through my system, and I continued to throw up.

I wanted to throw her away and start over.

Years later, a massage therapist would tell me that's because I'm a Leo. "In the wild, a mother lion would just leave a sick cub to die and let Mother Nature take its course," she said rubbing oil on my shoulders. "It's a natural Leo response."

Yeah, right.

For the rest of that first day, Lee visited the NICU and talked with doctors. When he came back to the room, he attempted to comfort me. Several times he tried to coax me into going back.

I couldn't. I wouldn't. I refused.

The next morning, that same perky nurse arrived, carrying a breast pump. With her bobbed hair bouncing, she explained how the two suction cups would be attached to my breasts, and told me I should try pumping every two hours until the milk came. I might have failed at the pregnancy part, but I knew from experience I could at least give her my milk. As soon as Tucker was born, before the cord was even cut, I'd put him to my breast, and he'd latched on immediately. I'd nursed him for a year.

After the nurse left, I pulled open my gown and followed the instructions. As the machine whirred, I stared at the television. The station flashed announcements about the hospital gift shop and the weekly menu from the cafeteria. I watched the screen until I had the gift shop hours memorized and knew the breakfast schedule for the next three days. I didn't make any milk.

When Lee came back from the NICU, he changed the channel. I tried pumping again. A documentary about Tasha Tudor came on. The narrator had a slow, deliberate voice. He described the life of the 80-something-year-old woman who'd written and illustrated over 80 children's books.

He said Tasha lived alone with her beloved Corgi dogs in a reproduction Cape her son had built in the hills of

Vermont. Every day, with her dogs at her heels, she walked a mile down her road and back again, just to retrieve her mail. She cut wood for her stove and dried herbs for savory meals. I could smell the boughs of lavender she collected from her garden. I felt the dewy grass and dirt road beneath her bare feet and saw blooming apple blossoms through her wrinkled eyes. Maybe Tasha Tudor wasn't telling me to go visit my baby, but she was giving me the strength to do so if I chose. She was showing me what a strong woman looked like.

✦

For two days, Lee continued to go back and forth to the NICU alone. He left Polaroids of Andie on my bedside table. I covered them with a box of tissues. On Wednesday morning, he was about to walk out the door when he turned and looked back at me. His eyes were red from lack of sleep and his hair was sticking up every which way. "You've got to see her at some point," he said and then walked out.

Fifteen minutes passed before I moved the box of tissues and picked up the Polaroids. It was hard to see her beneath all the tubes and wires, but when I held the photos at arm's length, I saw she was more human-like than I had thought. I ran my finger over her tiny fingers, her closed mouth. Her eyes were like the eyes of a baby robin I'd discovered as a girl in a fallen nest. Everything was there, just miniaturized.

When I looked up from the photos, Lee was standing in the doorway. "I had a vision," I told him. "I saw two paths. One leads to a funeral in a week. The other to a beautiful five-year-old girl." He stood still, watching me. "I'm going for the latter," I said.

Relief flooded his face and my journey as a NICU Mom had begun.

+

I believe in re-creating my own truth; that I can alter the memory of an event to fit the picture I wish I'd seen. In this memory, I imagine a kind old nurse, a Tasha Tudor–type woman, taking my hand. "Honey, I want you to be prepared for some things," she'd say gently. "First of all, many babies have been born this early. A micro-preemie, that's what we call them when they're this little." She'd point to the picture and say, "See how everything is there, just tinier? Tiny fingers, tiny toes, but a real baby? A real baby that just needs some time to grow. And lots of love." She'd smile down at me with her crinkly eyes, and I'd smile back. "That baby needs love from her Mama. I know you're scared, but deep down you have a lot of love for her. Deep down, it's there."

She'd ask me to close my eyes and see my love for my baby. With my eyes still closed, she'd tell me all about the NICU. "Neonatal Intensive Care Unit," she'd say, slowly and clearly. She'd tell me not to be afraid of the machines and noises. "They're just there to let us know your baby's doing okay." As she spoke, my body would relax. "We'd love to give you the chance to see her when you feel ready," she'd offer. "First, why don't you think of some things that you'd like to say to your new baby. Things she'd like to hear."

She'd hand me a thick sheet of ivory-colored notepaper

and a fine-tipped, black pen. When I looked unsure, she'd say, "You might want to tell her you're glad she's here. That you love her and know she's going to be healthy and strong." I would stare at the paper. "It won't be easy." She'd pat my arm, "But those words are what your baby will need to hear." She'd tell me to include a list of all the things I'd like to do with my daughter when she got older. "Like flying a kite at the beach," she'd say. "Or eating chocolate ice cream on a hot summer day." She'd squeeze my hand one last time, leaving me alone with my assignment. "Give me a call when you're ready to meet your baby," she'd tell me on her way out the door.

I still didn't want to see my daughter, but I knew it was time. I was too weak and sick to walk, so Lee eased me into a wheelchair and helped me put a robe over my hospital gown. I felt old. I looked down at the hospital-issued sock-slipper things on my feet. "Pathetic," I said and we laughed. The normalcy of laughter made me feel better. Lee stopped the wheelchair in the doorway. He squatted down in front of me, just like he would with Tucker. "You ready?" he asked. I wanted to weep. "Yes," I answered.

The journey to the NICU felt endless. We had to pass all the other maternity rooms filled with balloons, babies, and cheery parents; past the nursery filled with round bundles of joy, letting out healthy cries. I did not belong on that floor. I belonged with the guilt-ridden, terrified moms who didn't even feel like mothers.

An elevator took us to the sixth floor. The doors opened, and I saw the NICU ahead. Lee wheeled me to the front desk where he printed our names on a sign-in sheet. The receptionist picked up a phone and spoke to someone on the receiving end. "Andie's Mom and Dad are here." Suspicious that a phone call had to be made, I pictured scrambling doctors and nurses on the other side of the wall. "They're coming. Look busy over near their baby!" Lee, always able to read my reactions, smiled. "It's standard procedure," he said. We turned a corner and arrived in a small hallway with a sink where Lee showed me the proper hand-washing technique. Knowing what waited on the other side of that door, I took quite a while washing my hands. Lee finally reached over and shut off the water.

I felt hollow and shaky and slouched down in the wheelchair, willing myself to disappear. Lee opened the door. It took a moment to adjust to the glaring, overhead lights. Cutouts of pilgrims and smiling turkeys were still taped to the walls. At the nurse's station, several nurses turned from their paperwork to look in our direction. I turned away. I could hear what they were thinking, *There she is. That woman who hasn't even come to see her poor baby.*

We moved forward into a large, open room marked "NICU B." The incessant beeping of alarms, the florescent lights, and the bustling bevy of doctors and nurses felt overwhelming. The room smelled of hand sanitizer and fear. The six separate sections for each baby reminded me of stalls in a barn. Five of them were filled. As I passed the other babies, I wanted to look at them, to speak to their parents. "What happened?" I wanted to ask. But I knew not to look. Lee had cautioned me on the way to the NICU about the hospital's privacy rights. We had to pretend those other babies didn't exist. We had to ignore the parents, probably the only other people on Earth who could understand how we were feeling.

Andie was in the last station on the right, near the window. I expected to find her in the same plastic incubator I'd seen her in on the morning she was born. Instead, she was on a flat, open table lying limply on her back with bright, blue lights shining directly on her from above. A strip of white cotton was taped over her eyes. She wore the world's tiniest diaper and nothing else but wires and tubes. I could see the blue veins running beneath her papery, see-through skin. A pudgy nurse was standing near her station, writing on a chart. She looked up as we approached. "We saved the window view for this one," she said. I didn't smile, and she walked away.

Lee pointed to the lights. "She's jaundiced. The lights are supposed to bring down her bilirubin levels." He gazed down at her. "She'll be back in the isolette once those levels are normal."

From my wheelchair, I looked at her. The isolette had kept her at a safe, untouchable distance. Now that she was on the table, I could have reached out and touched her. I didn't. I studied her as though viewing an unusual artifact in a museum. I couldn't believe this creature had come out of my body.

Lee reached forward and with the tip of his index finger gently stroked her head, which was not much bigger than a plum. I watched his finger move slowly back and forth. She looked better than the Polaroids I'd seen. She really was all there. Ten fingers, ten toes. Her fingers were long, like mine.

Rising from the wheelchair, I took two steps forward. The pudgy nurse, who'd been watching us from across the room, flew over. I assumed she was coming to assist me. Instead, she berated me for my lack of shoes.

"With just those slippers on," she scolded, "any stray needle could stick your foot."

I sat back down in the wheelchair, too scared to move. Lee looked defeated. The nurse went back across the room, but I could feel her still monitoring my movements. "I want to leave," I whispered. Lee glanced at the nurse and nodded. He went around behind me, and took off the wheelchair brake, but before he turned I put my hand over his. Standing up quickly, I leaned over the tiny body. "Goodbye Andie," I whispered. "I'll be back later." And as I sat down, I knew I would.

As Lee wheeled me to my room, he told me about the conversations he'd had with the doctors. He spoke of medicines, machines, and enrolling Andie in some brain study because of a brain bleed. He had no idea that I wasn't really listening to anything he said. I was just relieved to be out of there.

Because of the caesarean delivery, we were due to stay in the hospital until Friday. I couldn't wait to get home. In the meantime, Lee phoned the office several times each day and worked toward completing his pending MBA project. It would have been crazy for him to quit at that point, when he had only two weeks left of an arduous last semester. We couldn't imagine when he'd find the time to finish if he stopped now.

So all week Lee stayed on the computer, and I stayed on the breast pump, still not making any milk. Twice a day I went to visit Andie, once in the morning and once in the afternoon.

Friday finally arrived. Our attempts to create comfort meant there was a lot to pack including clothes, blankets, pillows, and robes, not to mention all the flowers.

My dad drove in to pick us up. By late afternoon, the car was packed, the room was empty, and we were ready to go. After one last visit to see Andie, we were out of there.

I walked into the NICU on my Dad's arm. Lee followed a couple of steps behind. When we got to Andie's corner of the room, I stood looking at her tiny toes, the rise and fall of her miniature chest, and her little palm curled into her neck. Looking down at that tape across her eyes and the lights glaring down at her jaundiced body, I felt a wave of emotion swell up from a place I hadn't known existed. I began to sob uncontrollably. "I can't leave her here," I said over and over again. "I can't leave my baby behind."

The amazing thing is, it was really me saying those words. *Me*. Not the emotionally controlled me who'd just gone through the motions, acting in a way I believed others thought I should. That me was standing with her jaw agape, staring at this utterly exposed, new, vulnerable self. Ignoring the old me, I let myself experience the depth of those feelings and said the words I should have said, but didn't know how to express when Andie first arrived. "I'm here, Andie. I love you." In that moment, the uncertainty I'd felt about my capacity as a mother was gone. I *was* a mother. This startling maternal protection had risen from my core.

I was the woman who would stand in front of a moving train to protect this newborn baby.

7

Wishes

✦

WHEN WE TURNED ONTO OUR STREET, I sat up. Up and down the street, windows glowed in the evening darkness. I imagined our neighbors inside their homes; dressing for a Friday night out, popping a bowl of popcorn for movie night, or curled up on a cozy chair with a paperback and a glass of wine. I sighed. Dad stopped in our driveway next to our Volvo wagon. Lee turned to look at me in the backseat and said, "We're home."

He put his arm around me as we walked up the back step to the kitchen. The smell of roasting meat met us at the door, and my stomach rumbled. Mom's red wool jacket hung over the back of a kitchen chair and three votives flickered around a bouquet in the center of the table. I looked around at the kitchen we'd created, the painted cabinets, the white farmer's sink, the Shaker-style table Lee's dad made as a wedding gift, and the floral loveseat in front of the fireplace.

"Boo!" Tucker shouted, jumping from behind the loveseat. He was in his soft red sleeper with the padded feet. "Get over here, you," I said. He came running, and I scooped him up in my arms. His diaper rustled as I squeezed him tight. I wanted to fold him up, put him in my pocket, and carry him everywhere I went. Mom came in and put an armful of folded laundry on the chair by the fire. Her eyes looked drained. She tucked some stray hair into her ponytail. "How you doin', Leebo?" She kissed Lee's cheek. "Hanging in there, Mare." Lee squeezed her hand, then took Tuck from my arms and sat down on the loveseat in front of the fire. My mom turned to me. When she put her hands on my shoulders to hug me, her eyes filled with tears. "Let me pour you a glass of wine." She pressed my hair down with her palm. "How about a bottle?" I asked, sitting down next to Lee and Tuck, and staring into the fire.

Dad opened a beer for Lee. Mom handed me a nearly full glass of wine. "You hungry?" I nodded. "Good. Pam and Tom brought over a beautiful dinner." I pictured our next-door neighbors, desperate to do something, cooking all day. Pans clanged and the smell in the air grew stronger as Mom pulled the meal out of the oven.

We held our plates in our laps and ate in front of the fire. Our forks and knives scraped against the china as we cut into tender ham and roasted potatoes. Looking at the white floral pattern around the edge of the plate, I remembered what an important decision I thought it was, picking out just the right dishes.

After we finished eating, Tucker crawled onto Lee's lap and fell asleep. My mom refilled my wine glass, and I sank back into the couch, closing my eyes. I was just dozing, when the phone startled me awake. Lee looked at his watch. "Probably your brother or sister," Mom said. Dad picked up the phone. "Headquarters," he smiled.

His smile faded as he listened. "Just a moment, doctor," he said. "She's right here." Reluctantly, I reached for the phone. My hand was shaking. I wished Lee would take the call, but he nodded to Tucker on his lap and shook his head.

I took a deep breath. The only words I heard were "emergency, surgery, lower intestine," and I sank to the floor. Lee quickly passed Tucker to my Mom and took the phone. I could tell by the way his face tightened that he was hearing the same words.

"We have to go back in," he said when he hung up. He headed to the back door and took his coat off the hook.

None of us moved.

"What's going on?" my dad asked.

Lee looked at me. "They found a hole in Andie's lower intestine." He clenched his fists at his side. "They're taking her immediately for surgery."

"Oh my God," my mother said. Tucker stirred in her arms.

"Kasey," Lee said. "We have to go. Now."

I sat on the floor by the fire, unable to move. My father walked toward Lee, approaching him carefully, as he might a wild animal. "Lee," he put a hand on his shoulder. "Let me drive you to the hospital. It's been a long day."

Lee stepped away from him. "No, Kasey and I need to go alone." He watched me.

Finally, I stood up. The rug beneath my feet felt like it was moving. I held onto the back of the chair. "We can't lose her," I said.

My dad looked down at his shoes.

"She can't die."

My mother squeezed Tucker closer. "She won't die," she said quietly.

"She can't." I stood looking at a glass vase on the coffee table. If I'd had enough energy, I might have smashed it against the wall. "I saw her. She was five years old. She was beautiful and healthy." I looked out the window, past my reflection, into the darkness. A tiny casket. Lee dressed in black. "No," I erased the vision from my mind and looked at Lee. "We can't lose her."

"We've gotta go, Kase." Lee drew his hand through his hair. "They've already taken her for surgery."

I kissed Tuck's forehead and pressed my face into my mother's cheek. My legs were unsteady when I walked across the room. I followed Lee outside.

"Lee," my dad called from the doorway. "Please drive carefully."

✦

On the way back into Boston, I sat silently in the passenger seat. I don't know where the idea came from, but I closed my eyes and visualized a bright, swirling blue light, like the northern lights, streaming down from the sky and straight into Andie's tiny belly. I silently called to my grandmother, my guardian angel, who had died when I was eleven, "Please help her through this." I also called on Daniel, whom I'd never met, but who Andie was now named after.

And just as I was finding strength in this, I realized Lee was sobbing. I opened my eyes. The streetlights lit up his streaked face. "Why?" he was asking. "Why? Why? Why?" But he wasn't asking me; he was chanting the word in rhythm to some power I couldn't see. With tears running down his face, he pounded the steering wheel. I worried he might drive off the road, but thought too much had already happened for that to be possible.

Until this point, Lee had been controlled, solid. Now, his hopelessness felt startling. I looked at his hands clinging to the steering wheel, and realized he needed my support. Reaching over, I put my hands on his back and saw the same healing light that poured into Andie, surrounding him. His crying softened. I kept my hands on him all the way there. Finally, we were turning off the exit, driving back to the hospital we'd left just hours before.

Actually, it wasn't the same hospital. The doctor told Lee that Andie had been transported in her isolette, across the sky bridge that connected Brigham and Women's to Children's Hospital next door. The new hospital was unfamiliar, confusing. "Where the hell am I supposed to park?" Lee yelled at no one. It was almost eleven, and there wasn't an attendant in sight.

"Screw it." He parked the car near the front entrance. The lobby was empty. Behind closed metal grates, the gift shop and sandwich shop were dark. A security guard came around a corner. "We need to get to the surgical unit," Lee said. We were directed down a long hallway to a set of elevators. Lee started to run. "Wait," I called. I could hardly walk. He ran back, grabbed my hand and pulled me down the hall. "Do you need a wheelchair?" There was a trace of annoyance in his voice. The incision on my stomach burned and my legs ached, but I told him I could make it.

On the second floor, a sign directed us to the surgical waiting area. *Is this it?* I wondered. *Does our story end here?*

We tried to pass through the set of double doors, but a man in green scrubs blocked our way. "Are you Andie's parents?" I felt myself go cold. Lee nodded. "I'm Dr. S." He shook Lee's hand, then mine. He was wearing wooden clogs and a funky bandana around his head. "I just operated on your daughter." I saw a gold bridge on his back teeth when he smiled. "The surgery was a success." Lee reached out and steadied himself on the door frame.

We stood in the doorway while the surgeon discussed the intricacies of the surgery. "Her intestines were so tiny." He pinched his thumb and finger together to show us a tiny stream of light. I imagined his big hands trying to operate on a rubbery toothpick. The new scar on my belly burned. I rubbed the spot higher up and further to the right, where Andie's scar would be.

The hole, he said, was in her ileum, the part that connects the small intestine to the large intestine. He'd made a loop out of her small intestine. The loop emerged through the right side of her belly, allowing her stool to collect in an exterior bag called an ostomy bag.

A long time ago at a dinner party, I'd sat next to a woman who'd bragged about sneaking alcohol into concerts. Her trick, she told the dinner guests, was to tie a wine sack around her waist and tell security it was an ostomy bag. Everyone had laughed but me because I hadn't been sure what an ostomy bag was. The story finally made sense. It still wasn't funny.

The pediatric surgeon was smiling proudly. *My daughter has an ostomy bag*, I thought. *And this is good news?* But it was. She was alive and the ostomy would later be reversed.

"We're so grateful," Lee said as he shook the doctor's hand again.

"Just doing my job." He told us Andie had been wheeled back across the sky bridge to her home in the NICU.

We must have gone to visit her that night, but if we did, I don't remember. I just remember passing the large fountain in the hospital lobby. The fountain was broken and empty of water so all the coins were just sitting on the bottom. I thought of all those people making wishes before they threw them and wondered how many of those wishes actually came true.

8

Milk

✦

WHEN I WOKE THE NEXT MORNING, Lee was sitting up in bed working on his computer. "Hi, sleepyhead," he said. I stretched and smiled, sliding my hand onto his waist. Then I remembered the hospital and my tiny baby in the NICU. I groaned and slithered back under the comforter. My body ached but I forced myself out of bed. I could hear Tucker in the kitchen with my parents. They were leaving the next day. Like Lee, my dad had to be back in the office on Monday morning. Lee's parents would come for the week to take their place.

In the kitchen, I popped a piece of waffle in my mouth from Tucker's high chair tray. I was starving. "Hi Mommy," he said. "Hi baby." I kissed him on the cheek. My dad put his arm around me. "How ya doin', Arnold?"

I rolled my eyes. He had been calling me Arnold since fifth grade when I'd imitated Arnold Horshack on *Welcome Back, Kotter.* "Okay," I told him.

"That baby's a fighter." He squeezed my shoulder. "She's gonna be alright."

Mom dropped a few more pieces of cut-up waffle on Tucker's tray. "Your friends in this town are wonderful," she said, rinsing her hands under the faucet. "Leslie Rich called and people have signed up to bring meals for the next three months. Dede got Tucker into daycare with Josie on Mondays and Wednesdays, and your friend Betsy has her sitter coming on Tuesdays and Fridays." I watched her pour herself another cup of coffee. "We just have to figure out something for Thursdays, so you can visit Andie everyday."

I watched Tucker dipping his waffles into a bowl of banana yogurt. *But I don't want to visit Andie every day.* I hated the thought of going back to that hospital. Nurses were caring for Andie around the clock. She was surrounded by the world's top doctors. What did they need me for? I kissed the top of Tucker's head and breathed in the smell of his sleepy hair. *This is the one who needs me.*

Before this, Tucker had only been to daycare at my gym for an hour or so and sometimes the boy next door would babysit when Lee and I went out for dinner or a movie. Otherwise, we were always together. Now I'd be an hour away from him for hours at a time. We wouldn't take our walks, visit the library for story hour, or stop at the playground where he ran around with other little kids. My heart ached. I didn't want to leave him behind.

But I did. On Monday morning, we started what would become our daily schedule. Lee went to work and visited the NICU during his lunch hour. Tucker went to daycare, and I went to the hospital. For the first few weeks, neighbors and friends took turns driving me because I wasn't allowed to drive after the caesarean.

At the hospital, I pumped in a room off the NICU waiting room where moms could seclude themselves to breast pump. The room wasn't much bigger than a handicapped bathroom, large enough for just a small couch and a side table. Needlepoint quotes hung on the walls that said things like, "Just be patient. God and the NICU staff aren't done with me yet."

In the center of the room was an industrial-powered breast pump; a simple square machine, erect and proud, balancing atop a base of metal wheels. The wheels allowed moms to move about the room while pumping. Like a dutiful dog, the pump followed me closely as I chose my ideal location. The pump I was given by the hospital to use at home was broken and made a horrible screeching sound at the end of every cycle. Finally, I took it back to the hospital where I traded it in for a new one. That took up half of my visiting time one day.

For weeks, I spent lonely hours hidden behind that locked door, with two suction cups attached to my impotent breasts. The room seemed to grow smaller and smaller, and I began to fear the pump would chase me out of there, laughing and jeering, calling me a failure of a mother. I was pumping eight times a day, including twice in the middle of the night. I dutifully recorded my pumping schedule in a journal and continued to write "no milk" after each entry. Not one drop of liquid emerged from my burning breasts.

I met with two different lactation consultants who urged me not to quit, insisting the milk would eventually come and stressing the importance of breastfeeding. I'd nursed Tucker for a year; I didn't need to be told the importance of breastfeeding. The nurses advised me to spend time with my miniature baby. They said I'd be so full of love and maternal emotion, my milk would surely flow. But the deep fear I felt in looking down at her, attached to tubes, wires and alarms, only caused my breasts and my heart to retract further.

Even though I knew that every time I went into that pumping room it would be in vain, I wanted the nurses, doctors, my husband, and *my baby* to know I'd keep trying.

I tried everything. I took a prescription drug that made my body break out in a red, bumpy rash. I tried to express my milk by hand. I tried meditation, brewer's yeast, a multitude of vitamins, and an herb called fenugreek, which ancient Greeks used to increase a new mother's milk flow. I even drank a pint of Guinness Irish stout every evening. It didn't make my milk flow, but it sure made me feel better.

Lee and everyone in our family began urging me to quit. They saw my devastation and knew how desperate I was to be successful. If I hadn't been able to carry Andie to full-term, at least I wanted to offer her sustenance.

Every time I visited the NICU, there seemed to be another mother checking in before me with a little cooler in tow. She'd whisk off to the NICU freezer to deposit her properly labeled glass bottles, filled with creamy, liquid gold. I'd look away and hang my head in shame. Desperate thoughts of stealing the milk swirled in my head. But I didn't want some strange woman's milk going into my baby's body. I wanted Andie to have *my* milk.

But she never would. On a cold day in December, about three weeks after her birth, I finally waved the white flag, admitted defeat, and gave up. It just wasn't going to happen. Of course, once I decided to quit, the doctors, nurses, and even the lactation consultants all began touting the amazing benefits of ready-made formula. I listened politely and nodded my head, wishing they'd all shut up and leave me alone.

9

Carousels

◆

W HEN ANDIE WAS ALMOST TWO WEEKS OLD,
my brother, John, and his girlfriend, Lollie, drove
up from Manhattan. I watched them walk across the driveway toward our back door. Still in their mid-twenties, they
were so young and such a long way off from anything having to do with babies. I worried that seeing Andie would
terrify them. As we drove into the hospital, I tried to prepare them as I wished someone had done for me. I described everything in detail, from the entrance routine to
the numerous machines, to what Andie looked liked and
how unbelievably small she was. But I knew words could
never capture the real-life image.

At the NICU, I signed us in, we washed our hands, and
I led them in to see Andie. I closely monitored their unsure smiles as they looked down at my baby. John blinked
hard several times. I knew he was forcing himself not to
look away. Lollie tried to smile, but couldn't pull it off. We
stood in silence around the isolette. Quotes and photos surrounded Andie. When her nurses suggested that I decorate
her isolette, I hung photos of our family and quotes like,
"Won't you come out into the garden, my roses would love
to meet you" and "Every blade of grass has its own angel that
leans over it and whispers, grow . . . grow," from *The Talmud*.

The nurses had also tried to enlighten me on the machines, medicines, and tubes keeping Andie alive, but I didn't want to know. Decorating the isolette made me happy. Medical information did not.

We were still standing and watching her, trying to think what to say, when a British doctor came up from behind and asked if I was the "mum." Turning to him, I almost laughed out loud. He looked like he'd just crawled out from under the bridge of *The Three Billy Goats Gruff*. His big nose and brown, crooked teeth stuck out from his impish face. I replied that yes, in fact, I was the "mum."

"Please ask your visitors to leave," he said. "I have a medical issue to discuss with you."

"But my brother and his girlfriend just got here from New York to meet . . ." I started to say, but John and Lollie were already halfway out the door.

I watched the doctor pick up Andie's medical chart. "You'll have to wait until my husband gets here," I said. "He's dealing with all the medical stuff."

"Well," the doctor snapped, glancing up from the chart. "I guess it's about time you stepped in and took some responsibility."

I stood up straighter, my cheeks stinging as if they'd just been slapped. I willed myself not to cry and looked him in the eye. I hated him fiercely.

"The ductus arteriosus vessel between your daughter's aorta and pulmonary artery is not constricting on its own," he said in his *Masterpiece Theatre* accent. Registering the confused look on my face, he began again. "The PDA vessel acts like a valve that allows blood to flow between the heart and lungs. It hasn't closed, so we need to go in and surgically close it."

I reached for the wall to hold myself up. He quickly placed a stool behind me and I collapsed. I saw a smidgen of sympathy in his troll-like eyes. "I can't keep going on this roller coaster ride," I said. "Up and down, good news, and bad news, hope and despair."

He listened, and then said simply, "So don't ride the roller coaster. Ride the carousel instead. Some days will be up, some days will be down, but you'll stay steady."

I assumed that as my baby struggled for life, I was required to ride along on these plummeting, stomach-churning rides. I didn't know, or believe, that riding the merry-go-round was an option. I didn't know calm and steady were choices in the midst of all the chaos and confusion.

I imagined handsome, painted horses slowly circling around and around on an old-fashioned carousel. I pictured myself reaching out for the golden ring, capturing it in my outstretched hand, and winning a free ride—a ride straight out of NICU hell and away from this doctor telling me more news I did not want to hear.

"This surgery is not an emergency," he said. "But we need to schedule it as soon as possible."

We had time to prepare, meet with doctors, and learn about the various ways they would cut into our daughter's tiny chest. We also had time to worry and wonder.

We found out, through the nurse's rumored whispers, that the drug given to Andie to close the PDA valve had most likely been the cause of the hole in her intestine. Not only did the valve *not* close, hence the upcoming surgery, but it had also caused the need for the prior surgery, in which we almost lost her.

Could she survive another surgery? Two in two weeks? She'd survived the first strike of lightning. What were the odds of her surviving a second?

At home that night, I couldn't breathe. The notion of Andie's looming surgery hung on the walls, clung to our skin, seeped into our lungs. Lee and my brother sat at the kitchen table, watching me pulling on my winter coat. "Where you going?" Lee asked.

"I gotta get out of here," I said, pulling up the zipper. "I'm going for a walk."

"I'll go with you." Lee got up from the table.

"No." I walked to the back door. "I wanna go alone."

Outside, an angry December snow attacked me from all sides, but I didn't go back in. I wanted the bitter cold to sink deeper into me. I wanted to become too numb to feel any pain. I walked as tears froze on my cheeks. I was alone and cold and scared. I stood in the middle of a road near our house and sobbed under a lamppost.

Out of the darkness, a figure emerged. It was my neighbor, Gary, who gardened and spent his summers on Martha's Vineyard. He was dressed in a down parka. A fur-lined hood protected his head, and his sandy beard covered his face. Deliberate in his walk, he met me face-to-face under the lamppost and without a word pulled me into a strong, comforting hug. My mind wondered what he was doing out on this stormy night, but my heart knew he'd come with a message: I wasn't alone.

♦

The surgery would be a success. We'd learn that the doctors who feared having to cut open Andie's chest would instead access the valve through what they called a "keyhole incision" under her left shoulder blade. She would not have to recover with a chest tube and would avoid greater risk of infection.

However, we didn't know this as we waited for an update back at Children's Hospital.

Once again, Andie had been wheeled across the sky bridge for surgery. This time, we accompanied the team who escorted her. In the NICU, I'd watched them prepare her for the move and was shocked to witness all that had to be done. Everyone worked quickly and deliberately, detaching her numerous monitors, her feeding tube, and IVs. They disconnected her breathing tube last. After the oxygen was removed, a young nurse held a mask with a manual pump over Andie's mouth.

As we followed the mobile team down numerous hallways, elevators and the sky bridge leading over to Children's Hospital, my frayed, edgy mind kept imagining the nurse tripping, the mask sailing out of her hands, and my baby gasping for life like a fish out of water.

Once we'd reached Children's, the surgical team whisked our baby away. We were led to the adjoining waiting room with its smell of fear, blaring television, and packaged chips lined up behind the vending machine glass. I'd one day learn how to use this waiting time in a positive, effective manner. But during that second surgery, we did nothing but sit and stare at the white walls.

A round-faced woman with silver shoulder-length hair had come into the room. "Are you here for Andie?" she asked. We sat up, replying, "Yes," simultaneously. She pulled up a chair. "My name is Beth." Her voice was tender and calm. "I was assigned by the hospital as your social worker." Her sea green sweater looked so soft I wanted to reach out and feel it. "How are you holding up?" She touched my knee, then looked at Lee.

Lee leaned back in his chair and exhaled. "We've had a lot going on," he said.

She folded her hands in the lap of her tweed skirt and nodded. "That's what I've heard."

She stayed with us until the surgery was over. We told her about Tucker, our house, and our lives before everything changed. As we sat and talked, I became less aware of time. And then a surgical nurse was standing in the doorway. The seconds it took for her to cross the room felt like hours. "A success," she said smiling. "She's in recovery and we'll let you know when we're ready to wheel her back."

We all stood. Beth hugged Lee, then me. "Call me anytime," she said before walking out. Lee pulled me to him. "She did it," he whispered into my hair. I wiped away my tears and nodded. "She's a strong baby," I said. But when we looked at each other, I saw little hope in his eyes and knew mine reflected the same.

1 0

Gifts

◆

A NDIE'S HEALTH remained fairly stable after the surgery to close the PDA valve, but we prepared ourselves
for the possibility of another stomach-churning drop possibly lurking around the corner.

A constant stream of lavishly-prepared meals flowed
through our front door. But I found the colorful vegetables
and perfectly cooked meats unappealing. It was the sweet
desserts that fueled me, allowed me to look like Super Mom.
The constant sugar buzz of cookies, cakes, and carbs, along
with an ongoing consumption of coffee, allowed me to func-
tion. I was like a wind-up toy, bouncing off walls and tables,
moving too fast in ways that looked awkward and frenzied.

If I stopped to think or possibly feel, I was afraid I'd never
start again. I'd taken that British doctor's advice, I wasn't on a
roller coaster anymore. I was riding the merry-go-round, but
at a mind-numbing speed. Life felt like a race. Every morning
the checkered flag waved, and I was off. The sitter arrived,
or I dropped Tucker at daycare, and then navigated the hour
commute into the city through morning traffic. Once parked
and actually in the NICU, I spent my time meeting with doctors, nurses, insurance managers, and anyone else who *wasn't
my child*. During whatever moments I had to spend with
Andie, I read her a book, sang her a song, or lightly rubbed

her back. I'd bought a mini-tape recorder, and Tucker and I had read our favorite stories into the tiny microphone. When we weren't there, Andie heard our voices reading *The Mitten*, *Adventures of Frog and Toad*, and *Goodnight Moon*. Before leaving her, I'd switch on the tape player and console myself that I was still sort of there.

I was always so conscious of time and the ensuing mad dash back to Tucker. Torn between two worlds, I was trying to do it all and be it all.

Christmas was approaching like an oncoming train, and as hard to avoid—that, and pregnant women. There seemed to be an exceptionally large number of pregnant women in Boston that year. Around every corner, emerged one more big-bellied gal, each just a little cuter than the last. I wanted to trip them as they casually walked past, swinging their holiday shopping bags. I wanted to spit at them and scream, "Do you even appreciate what you have?" Instead I just smiled, silently hating them, and hating myself even more.

Everywhere I turned were reminders of Christmas. Wreaths tied to front grills of passing cars. A huge imitation tree just inside the door of the hospital lobby. Empty boxes wrapped in bright red paper, tied with gold bows set carefully underneath. By mid-December, friends were offering to do our holiday shopping, hang wreaths from our doors, even get our Christmas tree. I was tired and defeated, my well nearly run dry, but I turned down their kind offers, determined to do it all myself and somehow fake my way through this holiday season.

My Aunt Harriet drove down to visit, bringing along Christmas cookie ingredients, holiday decorations, and offers to care for Tucker so he could have a break from daycare. She also wanted to take me shopping, and I was excited for the diversion.

The day came and we dropped Tuck at daycare, stopped by to see Andie, then headed for the stores. Parking was difficult. The stores were crowded. Loud, lively holiday music streamed from hidden speakers. Poinsettia and evergreens crowded the windows. The colors were too bright. I wanted to make the most of the outing and enjoy the self-granted reprieve, but I was shaken by real life.

In a gourmet grocery halfway between the hospital and home, Aunt Harriet and I began collecting novelties for gift baskets so Lee and I would have something to give our parents on Christmas morning. I filled the cart with exotic mustards, dipping sauces, dried fruits, and French chocolates. I was standing with a jar of toasted almonds in one hand and spiced pecans in the other, when I suddenly stopped.

And I mean, *really* stopped.

Not just in that moment, but in all the frantic moments leading up to that one. I stood, nuts in hand, suddenly present and highly aware. "What am I doing?" I asked out loud. My aunt and several shoppers turned my way. "I have to get out of here."

I wanted to be with my children. I wanted to be with *both* of my children. I knew that wasn't possible, so why wasn't I at least with one of them? What was I doing standing in a swarming store halfway between them both? I looked down at the nuts, dropped the bags in the cart, and walked out the door.

✦

Later that week, I studied a new Polaroid hanging above Andie's isolette. It was a photo of a red-suited Santa, standing next to Andie in her lucite hospital home. He was leaning in, tilting his head so that his snow-white hair and beard touched the side of her plastic box. Her eyes were closed as she lay below her tubes and wires, apparently sleeping through her first visit with jolly old Saint Nick.

For some reason, that photograph totally pissed me off. I understood the intention, but it felt all wrong; forced and fake, like one of those mean scenarios from a teen movie, where the high school quarterback asks the school nerd to the prom. Everyone knows it's a cruel joke, and they go along with it anyway.

Lee couldn't understand my rationale. "Let it go," he said. But I wanted to hurt that Santa, rip off his beard and shove it down his throat. At least I could rip up the picture. But Lee wouldn't let me. He made me promise not to damage it. "It just feels like someday it will be important," he said.

So I took the photo off the wall and put it facedown on the counter.

Years later, Andie began looking through the photo album from her stay in the hospital. She pulled a picture out of the album with surprise. "Santa came to visit me in the hospital?" She looked over at me. "Wait till Daddy hears this!" she said.

I could already see the smug smile on his face.

In the midst of all the Christmas commotion, Lee and

I received a special invitation to attend the Boston Pops Holiday Concert on Christmas Eve. Though it was tempting, we thought we should decline because both our parents were visiting. But our parents insisted we go. When we found out Symphony Hall was within walking distance of the hospital, we decided it was okay.

We dressed for the occasion. I wore black velvet and Lee looked handsome in a sport coat and holiday tie. Our parents smiled at us from the door. We were excited. We felt alive. We'd agreed not to exchange gifts, but on the drive in, Lee pulled a strand of pearls from his jacket pocket. I was stunned. Every gift Lee had ever given me came with an electric cord. I didn't know how to respond, but I'd seen enough holiday jewelry commercials to help me through. "Oh, Lee," I said, putting my hand over my mouth. Then it was my turn. I told him the set of golf clubs he'd been drooling over was at home in our garage. It was our own suburban version of "The Gift of the Magi."

I sat back in the passenger seat, fingering the pearls, imagining the day I would hand them down to Andie. She'd be a beautiful, grown woman, dressed all in white.

Before the Pops, we stopped at the hospital, walking in like celebrities with a joyful, infectious energy about us. In contrast, the NICU felt exceptionally quiet. There was a sobriety among the nurses and a hazy light to the air. Unaffected, we visited Andie as if there were a photographer present. Holding hands, we leaned into her isolette and read her a Christmas story. We were like actors on a set, gazing down at someone else's child. For once I didn't feel guilty.

It felt good to pretend. We needed to pretend. Kissing our tiny Christmas angel goodbye, we walked back out into the cold daylight. Within an hour, we were sipping champagne at Symphony Hall.

Driving home in peaceful reverie, we listened to Garrison Keillor on the radio. He was relaying the story of a mom trying to help her newly divorced daughter make it through the holidays. He paused and in his smooth, deep voice said, "There is no pain like that of your children over which you have no control." Lee squeezed my hand. We both repeated the line. We would quote it for years to come.

At home, Tucker was dressed in a button-down Oxford shirt and brown corduroys, ready for the Christmas Eve Nativity pageant. It was our annual visit to the church a hundred yards up the road. He was holding his "Baby Andie" doll.

Just before Christmas, Tucker had asked for a baby doll. He was a real truck guy, so that surprised us. But in his childhood brilliance, he'd figured out a way to meet his longing for his sister. *Why hadn't we thought of that?* we asked ourselves, and took Tuck to the toy store to pick out a doll. She was big and round, and looked nothing like his real sister, but he loved her and carried her everywhere. He'd put her down for naps in the bassinet, where the real Andie would someday sleep, and tell us with a finger held to his lips, "Shhh, da baby's seeping."

The Nativity pageant was sweet. Local children dressed up as angels, shepherds and stable animals. I didn't allow myself to feel sad at the sight of the healthy round baby Jesus on the altar.

After the service we stood in front of the chapel so Tucker could visit the crèche. He'd noticed the manger scene and was eager to get a closer look. As he was trying to climb the donkey, a family strolled over. Like so many other families in town, they'd delivered us several beautiful dinners. I felt indebted and unsure how to thank them and everyone else who was supporting us. I readied myself to begin an appreciative speech of thanks, but the mother of the family spoke first.

"We want to thank you," she said.

"*Thank us?*" I said.

She continued, "We want to thank you for sharing your experience with us, for being so open and allowing us to help."

I was speechless. She said they'd grown as a family by offering their support and being part of Andie's experience. In that moment of grace, I was both stunned and perplexed; my notion of giving and receiving turned on its head. I suddenly remembered riding the school bus in sixth grade. I was the last of two remaining students. The other kid was an intimidating eighth-grader named Michael. He moved from his seat in the back and sat down directly in front of me. Turning around, he looked at me. I looked away, embarrassed and unsure.

He continued to stare at me for a long time, and then said, "I think you're pretty."

I glanced up at him, trying to gauge whether he was teasing me or not. I couldn't decide. "No I'm not," I said in return.

He looked hurt and, before turning away, said, "You could have just said thank you."

We'd received so much when Andie was born. I had desperately wanted to say no to all of the gifts of kindness sent our way, feeling that we'd never be able to pay everyone back and express the depth of our appreciation. Yet standing there in front of the manger on Christmas Eve, I realized that by receiving with openness and gratitude, we were, in fact, giving in return.

✦

Christmas morning was solemn. We'd used up our suppressed joy the day before. But Santa had come, and we did our best to cheer on Tucker as he shot baskets at his new hoop and pressed the correct letter on the electronic alphabet board. As I was collecting wrapping paper scattered around the room, I stopped in front of the tree and stared at the tiny pink hat hanging from a hook on a middle branch. It was the hat Andie had worn the first few days after she was born. I touched it and Lee came up behind me, whispering, "She'll be here next Christmas," and taking my hand in his, he lead me into the kitchen where his mom had a beautiful breakfast waiting on the table.

I I

Dreams

✦

CHRISTMAS WAS OVER. Needles were falling off the tree, the refrigerator was full of leftovers we'd never eat, and the trash was overflowing with wrapping paper. *Why?* I wondered, looking around at the mess. *Why put ourselves through this?*

I wanted nothing but ordinary days. Days without disruption.

"Back up, buddy," I said, pulling on Tucker's ankles to slide him a few feet away from the TV. I went over to put the ornaments away in their boxes. With each ornament I took off, more needles fell, and I suddenly longed for my childhood Christmases, when everything magically appeared and disappeared. I'd put on my shiny patent leather shoes and plaid dress and read picture books under the dazzling tree. By New Year's the tree was gone, and our house looked normal again. There'd been no magic or mystery to this Christmas, just a lot of work.

The phone rang. I set down a paper chain Tuck made at daycare and went to the kitchen to answer it.

"Hello?"

"Have you guys given Jimmy any money?"

"Joe?" I asked.

"Yeah. Listen, bad news. Jimmy fell off the wagon."

Jimmy, our friend Joe's younger brother, was supposed to have started our upstairs renovation project in early December. "He's headed to rehab," Joe said. I studied the fine carpentry work Jimmy had done in our kitchen. "You guys better find somebody else to do the work."

That night, Lee and I sat at the kitchen table eating pizza and drinking bottles of beer with the Boston *Yellow Pages* spread out before us. We were on the "D"s when Lee slammed down the phone. "There's no way we're gonna find someone." He took a sip of his beer and wiped his mouth with the back of his hand. "That guy just told me anyone who can 'swing a hamma' is working on the Big Dig." The Boston public works project was months behind schedule and millions of dollars over budget, requiring every contractor in the area.

Lee set his beer on the table. "What are we gonna do?"

"We'll find someone." I tapped the phone book. "And if we don't, we can start in the summer or next fall. It's just a change of plans."

"I'm tired of our plans changing." Lee ran his hand through his hair and it stood straight up like he'd stuck his finger in a light socket.

✦

On Saturday, Lee and I took Tucker to a friend's house for an extra-long playdate, while we went into the hospital. Marcia, one of Andie's nurses, came over to the isolette. "Hey guys." She had little gold hoops in her ears that I guessed were a Christmas gift. "You recovered from the holidays?" she asked.

I pulled the blanket off Andie's isolette. "I'm glad it's over," I said, peeking in at Andie behind the plastic wall. She was asleep with her hand curled next to her head. "But now we've gotta find a contractor."

"For what?"

"We want to convert a couple of rooms upstairs into a master bedroom," Lee said. "But the guy we had lined up fell through."

"You guys know you can't do any house construction once Andie's home, right?" Marcia put her hands on top of the isolette. "Her lungs will be really susceptible. Paint fumes, carpet smells, dust, anything like that can put her back in the hospital."

Andie's chest rose and fell with each breath of intubated air. "I hadn't thought about that," Lee said.

"Yeah," Marcia tilted her head. "It's kind of now or never if you wanna get that work done."

We spent the next two days on the phone, listening to the same story: No one could take on the project on such short notice. On Sunday night, after putting Tuck to bed, Lee and I stood in the upstairs kitchen.

"You know, this project isn't that big." He opened and closed the doors of the old wooden cabinets. "We could gut this in a weekend." He ran his hand over the yellowed wallpaper and squatted down to examine the linoleum. "We could totally do this," he said.

I banged my head against the wall. "Please tell me this isn't happening."

Lee stood up and tapped the wall separating the apartment kitchen from the living room. "This wall is pretty thin," he said. "It would be a piece of cake to take down."

"Leebo," I folded my arms across my chest. "*When* would we get this done?"

"We'll have to do it at night and on weekends," he said. "It's either that or we have a kitchen in our upstairs for the next five years."

I covered my eyes with my hands.

Lee walked over and wrapped me in a hug. "We can do this," he kissed my ear. And we did.

We spent every moment we weren't in the hospital, or at work, or in the car, or caring for Tucker, dressed in dusty work clothes behind a sheet of plastic we'd used to seal off the rest of the upstairs.

Joe showed up the first weekend and helped Lee tear down the wall and ceiling and carry loads of debris to the dumpster in the driveway. Our neighbors, Michael and Jonny, arrived the following weekend with tool belts to help Lee frame the new wall between the bedroom and bathroom. They joked about who had the manlier tool belt. The next weekend, Michael helped Lee hang sheetrock on the ceiling. Every night after work, Lee sat on the floor and played with Tuck, then changed into his Carhartt's, pulled on his tool belt and headed upstairs. As he sawed boards for the trim around the windows, I put Tuck to bed, cleaned up from dinner, and changed into my dusty old jeans so I could help.

Most nights we climbed into bed after midnight. Lee made sure his alarm was set for 5:20, giving him enough time to catch the train into Boston. The circles under his eyes were turning a yellowish brown.

One night, when we were too wired to sleep, I studied his profile in the moonlight coming through the window. He blinked at the ceiling.

"You okay?" I asked.

"Yeah," he shoved his hands under his head.

I moved my head onto his chest, smelling the clean laundry and sawdust scent of his t-shirt. His heart was beating slow and strong in my ear. "What are you thinking about?"

"We had so many dreams," he sighed. "Now everything's changed."

I didn't say anything, afraid to move in case he stopped talking.

"What if we have a child who lives with us for the rest of our lives?" he asked. "What's gonna happen to us? How will we live like that? What about the traveling we wanted to do after the kids grew up?" He took in a big breath and let it out.

I rolled onto my stomach and watched him. "Nothing has to change."

"But it does," he looked at me. "Everything has already changed. Nothing is certain anymore."

"You know, babe, I feel like we were traveling on one road," I traced my finger in a straight line on the comforter. "And then we took this unplanned detour. The first road was straight and paved and we could see for miles. This road is windy and full of pot-holes."

Lee watched me.

"But who knows?" I said. "Maybe this road will circle

back to the same place, or take us some place even better."
He looked up at the ceiling again.

"I still don't want to tell anyone she had a brain bleed,"
he said.

I thought back to the week after Andie's birth when Lee
told me Andie had suffered a brain bleed; that we wouldn't
know the long-term effects until she was close to three years
old.

I leaned up on my elbow. "How come?"

"People will expect her to fail. If she trips or bumps into
a door or struggles with math, everyone will say 'Of course,
because she had a brain bleed.' Even if they don't mean to,
the intention could set her up to fail." He'd clenched his
hands into fists. "Just promise me you won't tell anyone," he
said. "Even our parents."

"I promise." I reached over and kneaded his fists apart.
"Now get some sleep."

He checked his alarm one last time and rolled onto his
side, facing me.

I was almost asleep when his voice startled me awake.
"Do you think we should see a therapist?"

"What?" I looked at him. "Why?"

"The NICU books say that most marriages suffer."

"Lee, I love the fact that I'm married to a man who is
suggesting therapy. But I don't want to sit in someone's office and *talk* about what we're going through, I just want to
survive what we're going through."

"I know," he brushed a strand of hair back from my eyes.
"I just don't want to become a statistic."

"We won't," I said, laying my head back down. "Anyway, when would we find time to sit in a therapist's office? I don't know if you noticed, but we're a little flat out."

Lee slid his arms around me and pulled me to him. "Yeah, we're a little flat out," he said into my neck. "But I want to make sure we stay okay."

"We're okay," I squeezed his hand.

"Yeah," he said. "We're okay."

12

Whispers

✦

O N   A N   E A R L Y   M O R N I N G in the middle of January, I pulled off my pajama bottoms to find a large circle of blood. "About the size of a coffee can lid," I told the nurse on the phone. Dr. Shah sent me for an ultrasound. I went to the appointment alone because Lee and Tuck were both home with a stomach bug. The imaging office was near the hospital, so I could visit Andie right after the appointment. As the procedure called for, I drank a gallon of water before I got to the office. By the time I got on the exam table, I was about to burst. I just wanted to get the exam done so I could finally pee.

The radiology technician had red hair that looked dyed and glasses that were too big for his face. "How ya doin' today?" he asked, all nonchalant, picking up a long plastic device that looked like it belonged in a porn movie. He rolled a condom-like thing down the shaft and squirted a big glob of gel on the end. "Let's just slide this in and have a look." While he inserted the hard, plastic device, he began making small talk. "Where ya from?" he asked.

"Outside of Syracuse."

He told me he had friends there. As he moved the plastic rod around the inside of my vagina we figured out that my parents used the dry cleaner his friends owned. I'd just begun telling him about the other cleaner in town that ruined one of my mom's favorite linen tablecloths when he said, "What is *that?*"

"What is *what?*" I asked.

"That mass," he said.

"What mass?" I asked.

He turned the small video screen so I could see the black and white picture.

"Right there," he pointed. "That mass, right there."

Like *I* should know. "Well, what do *you* think it is?" I asked.

"Well . . . it could be a tumor," he said, then added, "but totally treatable with chemotherapy."

I immediately saw myself dead and buried, Lee caring for two young children, one possibly with special needs. The mystery of Andie's early arrival had finally been solved. I had cancer.

He pulled out the rod. "Let me get someone else to have a look." He left me lying alone in the room. Suddenly my urge to pee didn't seem all that important.

The door flung open and a younger, female radiologist marched in, followed by the technician. She said hello, noted my tears, and looked at the picture still displayed on the screen. "Do you mind if I have a look?" she asked, touching the back of my hand. I nodded, and she slid the rod back in. We watched as the images began swirling on the screen. "How long ago did you deliver?" she asked.

"End of November," I said. "Six weeks ago."

"And are you enjoying having a new baby at home?" she asked.

"Well," I began, when the technician said, "There. Right there. Do you see that?" He put his finger on the monitor.

"I see it," she snapped at him.

She studied the screen while I held my breath

"It could be a fibroid," she said.

"I've never seen a fibroid that's looks like *that*," the technician said.

"Well I have," she shot back. "Listen," she said to me. "Why don't you get dressed. We'll give your doctor's office a call and you can take these films over to him."

I couldn't answer. I just nodded. The tears clinging to my chin fell to my chest.

When they walked out the door, I stayed on the table and stared at a long photo on the wall. It was a whole bunch of babies, about twenty of them, lined up shoulder-to-shoulder, all smiling at the camera. I thought about the hours and hours it must have taken to get that one stupid photo. "Fuck you," I said to the babies. I ripped off the paper gown, wiped the blood and gel mixture from between my legs and pulled on my black stretch pants and black turtleneck. As I was tying my boots, I realized that I wouldn't get to see Andie after all and began sobbing. I walked out of the office and sat on the bench in the hallway, crying and waiting for the films. The female doctor handed them to me without a word. I stood up to leave. "Are you okay to drive?" she asked.

"Yeah," I said.

Outside in the parking lot, I sat down on a curb and dialed home. When Lee answered, I whispered into the phone. "I might have cancer."

I thought of my friend Sue, whose son, Dominique, has

Down syndrome. A year after we'd met, she was diagnosed with breast cancer. "That's not fair," I said to her one morning over coffee. "You already had your thing when Dom was born with Downs."

She put down her coffee and said the words I'd remember long after she was gone. "Life don't work that way, girlfriend."

After I called Lee, I went to Dr. Shah's office for blood work. He was leaving the next day for a three-week trip home to India. As I left his office, he had already begun calling cancer specialists.

When I got home, we took a slow walk around the block. We'd been discussing the health of our daughter for so long, we never thought we'd be talking about mine. We walked mostly in silence until Lee leaned into me and whispered, "You can't leave me."

"I won't," I whispered back.

Dr. Shah called that night to tell me the plan. I pictured his wife at home, packing for their trip while he stayed late at work. He said a partner of his would take over while he was gone. While we waited for the results from the blood work, I'd have a D&C so the mass could be biopsied. A D&C (or Dilation and Curettage), means the cervix is dilated and the mass is surgically removed. Curettage means that a curette, or sharp surgical device, is used to scrape or scoop out tissue. *How fun.*

A few days later, I was in a hospital I'd never been to before, having the mass scraped out of my uterus by Dr. Shah's partner. I can't remember her name, but I do remember her soft brown curls and kind eyes. Several times I yelled out and squeezed Lee's hand. "Sorry," the doctor kept saying. "So sorry. But I really have to dig in there to get a good sample of the mass." When it was over, she said they'd try to get the biopsy results back as soon as possible.

In the days that followed, Lee went to work, Tuck went to daycare, and I went to the hospital. My daily visits with Andie were so important and they felt too short. I was angry and resentful about all the interruptions. Someone always needed to talk to me, and I just wanted to be alone with her so we could get to know each other. Andie's nurses offered me sad smiles. Lee talked to Fletcher about possible treatment options if the mass turned out to be cancer. Everyone in my family kept leaving phone messages asking if we'd heard anything. At night, Lee and I knelt next to Tucker's bed, studying his innocent face.

After almost a week, the doctor called to say that the mass was a fibroid cyst. I did *not* have cancer.

The NICU nurses wanted to hunt that thoughtless technician down and castrate him. They wanted us to be pissed off, too, but I was too relieved to engage in those conversations. I didn't have cancer. That was redemption enough. I'd done a lot of soul searching during that long week, and had been asking myself some serious questions, mainly, *What the hell am I doing?*

The scare had brought my perpetual adrenaline rush to a screeching halt. I was tired, deeply tired, and no amount of sugar or caffeine was going to lift me. My time with Andie was suddenly sacred. I had been given a gift—an incredible gift. My life. My daughter's life. My son's. My husband's. I was finally able to see just how blessed I was.

13

Healers

✦

THE CANCER SCARE sucked out the last of my reserves, and I was running on empty. Tucker, Lee, and I needed a day of rest at home together. We decided we'd visit the hospital just once on weekends. Even though Andie's health was more stable, I still felt guilty not visiting every day. But her nurses insisted we take care of ourselves and assured us they'd give Andie lots of affection when we weren't there. We called them her "NICU mommies."

She had four primary nurses—Yvonne and Marcia, who worked the twelve-hour day shifts, and Tina and Janice, who worked the same shifts at night. Yvonne, a small sprite-like woman probably in her late sixties, hadn't originally been assigned to Andie, but she'd traded with another nurse. She was known in the NICU for working with the scared teenage moms. Yvonne had faint wrinkles sketched into her delicate features, and when she spoke, I wanted to curl up in her lap and let her pat my head, imagining she would say, "Shhh. It's okay. This little baby's gonna be just fine." I realized later she was the Tasha Tudor nurse I'd been looking for all along.

Marcia lived only a few towns over from us with her husband and three kids. When she laughed, she covered her mouth with her hand and her eyes crinkled in the corners.

I loved to make her giggle. One day, I came in with a new haircut that made my messy blond hair look like it had never been brushed. When I told her the cut was called the "Bed Head," she laughed so hard she bent over and slapped her thigh. "You are so funny," she said. "I'm gonna miss you when that baby goes home." During her day shifts, Marcia complained Andie's hair stood straight up. She was always trying to smooth it down with her fingertips. Marcia told me that one morning, when Janice was passing her Andie's report, Marcia had mentioned her ongoing battle with Andie's hair. "Oh, that's me," Janice said. "I put a little dab of surgical gel in her hair and give her a mini-Mohawk."

We never saw Janice and Tina, Andie's night nurses. But they'd taken Polaroids of themselves with Andie and taped them around her isolette. Janice had been the one who saved Andie's life by noticing her distended belly. Shortly after Andie was discharged, I found out Janice left the NICU because she was diagnosed with breast cancer.

Lee often talked with Tina on his nightly calls to the hospital. After hanging up, he'd lie comfortably back in bed. "She's wonderful," he'd say.

From the Polaroids, I saw Tina had shoulder-length brown hair, dimpled cheeks, and a beaming smile. Marcia told me Tina had a new baby girl of her own at home. Years later, we gave Andie a fuzzy, stuffed lamb for her fourth birthday. "Does the lamby have a name?" I asked.

"Yeah," she said, like she'd known before she opened it. "Tina."

✦

At home, I began nurturing myself more. I ate healthier foods, took naps, read books, and listened to music. Just little bits here and there, but enough to start refilling my dry, thirsty well. I was turning inward, not answering the phone as much, and discouraging visitors. I needed quiet, uninterrupted peace.

One Thursday afternoon in late January I didn't go to the hospital, and Tuck and I spent the day at home, never changing out of our pajamas. While Tuck was napping, I looked out at the sun reflecting brightly off the snow outside. Drawn by the light, I wrapped myself in a long winter coat, grabbed my book, and went to sit on the front porch rocker. I was reading Barbara Kingsolver's *Prodigal Summer*. It was a diversion, an escape from my everyday life. I would have leapt into the book if possible. I'd been reading for a little while when a red minivan pulled into the driveway. I wanted to duck down and disappear, but there was nowhere to hide. "Damn it." I set my book down.

Joan, the mom of one of my writing students, got out of the van and stood at the edge of the lawn. I hadn't seen her since I'd cancelled my after-school writing workshops. A stretch of snow separated the porch and driveway. She could have crossed it, but must have sensed my unwelcoming mood.

"I just stopped to see how you're doing." She looked thinner than I remembered and her short brown hair showed silver at the roots.

"Oh, I'm fine," I lied. *Go away. Go away. Go away.*

She hesitated, then asked, "How are you *really* feeling?"

"*Really* feeling?" I asked. Did she *really* want to know? So I stood on my front porch and told her that I felt lost and removed from life, like I was floating. I told her about the constant feeling of panic living just below the surface of my skin. She didn't back away. She didn't jump in her car and drive off. Instead, she asked if I was "seeing" anyone. I knew she meant a therapist and I told her what I told Lee, that I didn't want to sit in someone's office and talk about how I was feeling, I wanted to stop feeling.

She said she knew a woman who might be able to help us. "She's an energy healer."

"A what?" I asked.

"An energy healer. It's like an active form of therapy. It's really powerful and works on many levels. I have her card if you want it."

I thought if I took the card, I could get rid of Joan, so I said sure.

She reached in her car and took a few steps across the snow toward the porch. I took a few steps off the porch and met her halfway, grateful this interruption was about to end.

I looked down at the fine black script on the card. *Karen McCarthy*. "How do you know her?"

"Someone gave me her name a few months ago," she said. "I don't know if you heard, but I was diagnosed with breast cancer."

I looked up. "No, I hadn't heard." My Aunt Mimi's favorite line rang through my head. *Well, enough about me. Let's talk about you. How do you feel about me?* I wanted to reach out to her, but how could I pretend I hadn't put up an invisible force field, hoping she'd go away? *Hey, Joan, now that I know you have cancer, how about coming in for a cup of tea?*

"I'm sorry," I said. She shared a few details about her illness while we stood awkwardly sinking into the snow, knowing there was so much more to say.

"Thanks for the card," I stepped back on the porch. "I'll call her."

I watched Joan drive off. Looking again at the card, I felt myself shiver.

Then I walked in the house and picked up the phone.

◆

Later that week, a neighbor watched Tuck while Lee and I went to our first appointment with Karen McCarthy. It was early evening and the snow looked blue in the dim light. On the drive there, Lee kept switching radio stations. "Stop it," I said.

"What are we going to do there?" He was still pressing the buttons.

"I don't know," I said. "We'll just check it out. If it's totally weird, we won't go again."

When I made the appointment, I'd asked Karen to tell me a little about energy healing. "Everything is energy," she said. "Humans are made up of energy, and in the human system, when energy gets blocked or stops moving, the result is illness and disease." She went on to explain that we weren't just physical bodies; we had mental, emotional, and spiritual levels as well. In order for true healing to occur, we had to heal on all of those levels.

I hadn't understood what she was talking about, so I told

Lee it was a mind-body sort of thing. Although we felt anxious and unsure about the appointment, our uncertainty was trumped by defeat and exhaustion. We'd try anything as long as it didn't take too much time away from our children. Karen's house was just fifteen minutes away from ours. It was red and sat among other nice homes on a tree-lined street. A sign on the door welcomed us and asked that we remove our shoes. The Berber carpet on the stairs leading down to the office felt soft and giving under our stocking feet. At the bottom of the stairs, the door marked "OFFICE" was closed. We held hands on the couch in the large waiting area with its overflowing bookshelves and big bin of toys. We could hear muffled voices on the other side, and then a loud burst of laughter. The door opened. "Alright, my dear. Great work today," we heard.

Two women emerged, one headed for the stairs, and the other turned to us. "You must be Lee and Kasey." She was about five foot eight inches, my height, with bangs and thick, brown hair that fell to her shoulders. She wore khaki pants and a turtleneck sweater. She looked so . . . *normal*. We stood and shook hands. I knew Lee would like her firm handshake. As she led us into her office, I realized I'd been expecting someone more like our hippyish birthing class teacher. I thought there'd be incense, tapestries, and candles. When I got to know Karen better, I told her how shocked I'd been by how normal she looked. She laughed. "My friends call me Glenda the good witch," she'd said.

We sat on plaid cushions in straight-backed chairs across from her desk. I glanced at the massage table to my right and then tilted my head to read the titles on the long white bookshelf above her desk. *You Can Heal Yourself* by Louise Hay, *Everybody's Guide to Homeopathic Medicines,* and *Gray's Anatomy.* A tall skeleton watched me from the corner; it was dressed in a fleece scarf and hat. Her office felt safe and comfortable. She poured us water from a jug and asked us to tell her our story. Lee stayed quiet. I took the cue and spilled our tale into the room. Every time I told Andie's story, I gained some temporary breathing space. The story was finally outside of me, rather than in.

"It sounds like you guys have a lot on your plate," she said. She spoke in a clear, direct manner. It was the voice I'd been searching for. She talked about caring for ourselves first in order to best take care of our children. She used the analogy of oxygen on a plane. "When the masks fall down," she said, "Mom and dad have to take care of themselves first, or they're useless to their children." Within our bodies, she explained, there exist a series of pathways called meridians through which energy travels like a circuit, conducting electricity. According to Karen, blocks in these energy fields result in bodily dysfunction. Throughout that first meeting, she stressed the importance of drinking water. "If you're made up of energy, or electricity, what does it conduct through best?" Of course the answer was water. Without enough water, the energy can't move and gets stuck.

She also gave us a series of exercises called Brain Gym to help calm and center ourselves. Developed by Dr. Paul Dennison, the exercises worked by utilizing both sides of the brain, crossing the center meridian or the mid-line of the body. They were surprisingly simple and took just a couple of minutes. One involved just crossing an opposite hand to the opposite knee. Although quick and simple, the exercises were incredibly calming.

Near the end of the appointment, I told Karen about my Christmas shopping experience, when I'd found myself between both children, but not with either. I told her how guilty I felt when I wasn't with them. "You don't need to worry about that," Karen said. "You have an energy field that protects your children even when you're not with them."

"Really?"

"Absolutely."

I wanted to ask more questions, ask her to explain how she knew that. But instead I leaned back in my chair, let out a big breath, and felt my shoulders release. I hoped her words were true because they flooded me with relief and comfort.

14

Angels

✦

IN LATE JANUARY, a big snowstorm hit the Boston area. Big, I should say, in the eyes of Bostonians. As a native of upstate New York, my childhood memories are dominated by blizzards, and I was always amazed at the local reaction to these seemingly infrequent storms. While others were in storm panic, I stuck to my routine, dropping Tuck at daycare and driving into the hospital for my morning visit with Andie. Schools must have been closed, because there was little traffic for most of my drive. But when I got near the hospital, the storm's effect became clear. Traffic crawled. Horns blared. Cars sat in the middle of intersections, stopping traffic in every direction.

I looked over at an elderly couple, stuck in a car to my left. They were obviously as determined to get to their morning appointment as I was. I wondered what their appointment was for. Was she sick? Was he? Were they visiting an ailing loved one? What was their story?

As we crept ahead, our two lanes became one, and I let the elderly couple go first. A cop was directing traffic in front of the hospital's parking garage, and the couple stopped and rolled down their window to talk to him. I didn't hear the exchange, but when their car veered away from the garage I thought, *Uh oh*.

Pulling up, I rolled down my window.

"Garage's closed," the cop said in his thick Boston accent.

"Where am I supposed to park?" I quickly calculated how little time I had left to visit Andie.

"Don't know what to tell ya." An overcoat hid his badge, but I imagined his name was Sergeant O'Sullivan or Officer McNally.

I sighed. Before rolling up my window, I said aloud, mostly to myself, "I just wanted to see my baby."

The cop's blue eyes looked out from under the stiff brim of his black cap. "How long ya gonna be?" he asked.

"How long can I be?" I asked.

"Tell ya what." He glanced at the cars trailing past. "If you're not too long, you can pull over right here and I'll watch your car for ya." He pointed to a street corner that had been plowed, but wasn't really a parking space.

I almost asked him if he was sure, but I didn't dare. Instead, I promised him I'd take just a half hour to visit. He nodded and waved me on. He had a fine-looking smile.

Because every minute was precious, I ran as fast as I could up to the NICU. Even though the visit was condensed, I was able to read Andie two stories and tell her all about the newly fallen snow.

Running back down, I called Lee from my cell phone and told him my story. He suggested I buy the cop a cup of coffee.

Down on the street everything was just as I'd left it. Traffic was still stopped and desperate drivers were being turned away from the garage. My gray Volvo wagon was still parked at the corner.

"Hi!" the cop called over when he saw me. Snow swirled around him. "I had to fight tooth and nail to protect that car. The meter maids were all over it, trying to ticket, wanting to tow." He gave me his big dimpled smile.

"I can't thank you enough," I told him. "Can I at least run in and buy you a cup of hot coffee?"

He waved at me. "Nah," he said. "That's awful nice of you, but I'm good."

"You were my angel today."

He winked at me. "Hey," he called as I was walking away. "What's your daughter's name?"

"Andie," I called back.

He nodded.

I was about to get in the car when I hesitated. "What's yours?"

"Andy."

I can still feel the shivers running down my spine.

I smiled the whole way home, filled with a deep sense of knowing, a knowing that there was something so much bigger at work than I could ever imagine.

15

Airplanes

✦

"I wish I wasn't so far away," my sister, Libbie, told me on the phone one night while I was spooning pasta onto plates. "I can't wait to see her again." Libbie had been able to visit for a few days after Andie was born.

"When you come, we'll look for your wedding dress. The big day's gonna be here before you know it." She was getting married in June near her house in Colorado. "I'll call the shops, and we'll make a girl's day of it."

Libbie and I talked at least once a day. She was the one person, besides Lee, who I really opened to. As I put the plates down on the table, I pictured Lib and myself dressed up, walking into boutiques on Newbury Street, lunching on crisp salads, and sipping wine at linen-covered tables.

A couple of days before Libbie was to arrive, the doctors moved Andie to an intermediate room in the NICU. She'd gone from a formal dining room to a tavern. This room was casual and at ease, filled with healthier, bigger babies (if you consider three pounds bigger). They slept in plastic, open-air cribs and alarms didn't sound every minute. The air wasn't as desperate. If we wanted, we could pick her up and rock her in the glider without asking a nurse for permission.

"Colorado looks good on you," I told Lib as I steered

the car out of Logan Airport's parking area. After college, she moved out to Vail for the ski season and never came back. She'd gone from ski bum to manager of a luxury hotel, and now she looked fit. There were streaks of blond in her shoulder-length hair.

We went straight to the hospital to see Andie, and when we walked into Andie's new room, Libbie seemed to know right where to go. I followed *her* as she led the way to Andie's station. "Hi Andie Lou." She looked into the crib and gently stroked Andie's cheek with the back of her finger. When Andie woke up Libbie reached right in and picked her up. I looked around to see if a nurse was nearby in case we needed help. But Libbie didn't need help. She brought Andie up and gazed deeply into her eyes. Andie looked right back at her. I sat down in the glider, feeling like a third wheel and wondering if Libbie had been Andie's mother in a past life. I fantasized Lib would move back from Colorado and help me raise her. She could give her the love I couldn't.

For the millionth time, I wished I'd played with dolls when I was little, then I might have been a more natural mother. Libbie played with dolls. Tucker was home playing with his baby doll. It seemed like everyone wanted to care for babies but me. Of all the people to be stuck spending hours in a hospital ward filled with sick babies, I never imagined I would be one of them.

Libbie put Andie down, and I stood up to join her at the crib. We looked down at her. She was dressed in the little pink-and-white striped preemie one-piece I loved. "Do you want her?" I asked.

Libbie laughed. "I'd take her in a minute," she said.

Marcia came into the room. "I put her in your favorite outfit for your sister." She tucked a pen behind her ear.

"Thanks, Marcia," I said. "This is Libbie."

"Nice to meet you." Marcia shook Libbie's hand. "We love your little niece."

"So do I," Libbie said. They chatted about Lib's trip east. I told Marcia about our wedding dress shopping plans.

"Oh, you're getting married?"

Libbie held out her hand to show Marcia her engagement ring.

"Where's the wedding?"

"Colorado," Libbie said.

"When?" Marcia asked.

"June." Lib glanced down at Andie, sucking on her big blue pacifier. "So we've got to get this little one healthy before then, she's got a big wedding to go to."

Marcia fumbled with her clipboard. She was frowning. "What's the matter?" I asked.

"I hate to tell you this." She tugged on her earlobe. "But an airplane's the last place you want that baby. It's a haven for germs and sickness."

Libbie and I looked at each other. I covered my eyes with my fingers, trying to push the tears back in.

"I'm so sorry," Marcia said.

✦

"We have to postpone the wedding," Libbie said over lunch. There were no linen tablecloths, white wine, or sprigs of white roses. Instead, we sat at a tall wooden table in the bar of a Mexican restaurant, drinking margaritas and sharing fajitas. We both wore the little black cowboy hats they passed out with the kid's meals.

"You're not postponing the wedding," I said. "Even if you postpone it, she still won't be able to get on a plane for who knows how long."

"Well, what are we going to do?" she asked.

I looked into my little sister's worried brown eyes and said, "For now, we'll do the only thing we can do . . . *drink.*"

We clinked our glasses.

"To our girl's day," she said.

"To our girl's day," I repeated, and we both took a big sip of our drinks.

During her visit Libbie wanted to spend most of her time at the hospital with Andie or home with Tuck. We did wind up finding her a wedding dress at a small boutique not far from our house. I hadn't even known about the shop until a neighbor mentioned it. We drove over one late afternoon with Tucker in the back of the car. A carefully groomed older man met us at the door. After Libbie explained the circumstances and why we didn't have an appointment, he put his hands on his thin hips and said, "Doll, rest assured. Freddie is here to help you. I am going to find you the perfect dress." And he did. It took a few tries, but when he found the dress, we all knew it. Libbie's olive skin glowed in the ivory strapless gown. I pulled out my cell phone and called my mom to report our success. After I hung up I realized Tucker had snuck away. Libbie and I searched the racks of white gowns calling his name. Finally, we turned a corner and found him standing in his denim overalls, hugging a child-sized mannequin dressed in a puffy, white flower girl dress. "Mommy," he said. "I found an angel."

◆

The morning Libby left, Tucker and I drove her to the airport shuttle bus. "I don't want to leave," she said. When she squeezed Tucker in one last hug, her tears dripped into his hair. "I'll come back as soon as I can." She handed Tuck to me.

"I know you will," I said. I shifted Tucker onto my hip and tried to smile as I watched her wheel her suitcase toward the bus. Tuck and I stood on the sidewalk and waved until the bus pulled out, and we could no longer see Libbie in the window.

I cried the whole way home. Then I took Tuck to daycare and drove into the hospital.

16

Breath

✦

I WALKED INTO THE NICU to find Andie's nurse, Yvonne, sitting in the glider with Andie in her arms. On the table next to her blue pacifier sat a little bottle filled with thick formula. All the preemies were given pacifiers because they had to learn the mechanics of sucking. "It's time to teach this little one to eat," Yvonne said in her grandmotherly voice. "You ready to try?"

I'd nursed Tuck for so long, I didn't really know how to feed a baby a bottle. I looked at Andie, resting comfortably in the crook of Yvonne's thin arm, with the feeding tube still in her nose. "No, you go ahead." I pulled a chair up next to Yvonne and watched her coax the nipple of the bottle between Andie's pink lips. Andie sucked a few times then stopped. She started and stopped several times. Yvonne looked at me. "She's getting it," she said. "It takes a while for them to figure out the mechanics of sucking from an actual bottle." Yvonne jiggled the bottle a bit and Andie started sucking again. I looked at the clock on the wall.

"Here, you give it a try," Yvonne suddenly put Andie in my arms. She handed me the bottle. I shifted Andie, worrying I'd drop her. Yvonne stood up. "Okay," I said, unsure. "Here you go, Andie." And when I pushed the nipple between her lips, she started sucking! I looked up at Yvonne, and she smiled. Then she walked to the other side of the room to check on the other babies. Leaning back in the glider, I felt the warmth of Andie's head in the crook of my arm and closed my eyes. When I opened them, Andie had stopped sucking. I jiggled the bottle, but she didn't respond. Her face was turning gray. I stood up. "Yvonne," I hollered. Yvonne ran across the room, her yellow scrub coat flying behind her. "Okay, now," she said, taking Andie out of my arms and blowing into her face. "Wake up, you," she shook her up and down lightly. I watched Andie's eyes fly open. I thought I was going to throw up.

Yvonne put her down in the crib. "I think that's enough for her first time," she said. I held onto the edge of the crib. "What just happened?" I asked. Yvonne patted my hand. "It was just a bout of apnea," she said. "She gets sleepy and stops eating and then forgets to breathe. We just have to remind her." I looked down at Andie. When I touched her cheek, I saw my hand was shaking. "You'll get used to it," Yvonne said.

But I never did. I was so scared every time I fed Andie that I asked a nurse to sit at my side throughout the entire feeding. Every time Andie stopped breathing, so did I, and the nurse would have to take over.

I had mixed feelings about caring for Andie. I wanted to feel more like her real mom, and yet I was unsure of my ability to take care of her. But I was becoming jealous of the nurses and all the time they spent with Andie. One morning I found a new Polaroid of Andie and her night nurse, Janice. Janice had stuck the picture inside Andie's crib, right next to her head. I felt silly, but I was upset. It was one thing to tape a picture on the wall, but to put it right in her crib crossed some line I didn't even know I'd drawn. I took the picture out, taped it to the wall and said to Andie, "If anyone's picture is gonna be in that crib with you, it's mine."

I was slowly becoming more comfortable taking care of her, but if I ran into trouble there was always a nurse nearby, ready to rescue me.

Then one morning Andie's doctor was waiting by her crib when I arrived. "Good news," she said, tapping the side of the crib. "This one's almost ready to go home."

"Home?" I asked. "Whose home?" We'd been so concerned about Andie's survival I'd kind of forgotten she'd actually come home. "I'm not a nurse," I said to the doctor.

She laughed. "You don't need to be a nurse," she said. "We'll make arrangements soon," she told me. And then she walked away.

I looked around at the nurses bustling around the room. *This is our home*, I thought. I'd gotten used to the NICU; it had become my life. I knew all the guys in the parking garage and fantasized about running away with the flirty one who had a pierced eyebrow, shaved head, and sexy smile. The two cashiers at the coffee shop were my pals. They knew I liked lots of cream in my hazelnut coffee. How could I leave the big goldfish tanks, the tile bathrooms, and the bitchy receptionist, Zelda? How could I leave the nurses? I needed the nurses. Andie needed the nurses.

When Andie was first born, we were told she'd probably go home about a month after her original due date. "Shoot for Easter," a doctor had said. Easter fell in mid-April. It was early February, and this doctor was telling me Andie was ready to go home. Was she out of her mind? How could she even think about sending this vulnerable little baby home? I looked down at Andie, asleep in the crib. She had on a tiny preemie sleeper with purple flowers on it that was way too big for her. I pictured Andie's face turning gray every time she stopped breathing during her feedings. That doctor didn't know what she was talking about.

When I got home, Lee and I talked about whether the insurance company was pushing her early release. The medical expenses required for Andie's care were unfathomable. We'd received a bill for a week of her hospital stay, and when I saw the charge *I* stopped breathing. My breath returned when I called the insurance company and found out the bill was sent to us in error. During my moments of deepest despair, I consoled myself that at least we didn't have financial worries. That's not to say my daily trips to the hospital and Lee's noontime cab rides weren't eating into our budget. Gas, parking, and hospital meals all added up to quite an expense. We'd started calling Andie "the million dollar baby." But we weren't in the same boat as the families with preemies we'd seen on a video in one of the NICU family rooms. A lot of parents without medical insurance had lost their homes, businesses, and everything they owned to pay the bills required to keep their babies alive. A doctor friend told us that when the insurance company is billed, they negotiate with the hospital and pay a percentage of the total bill. If the bill is $10,000 they might pay $7,500. When an uninsured patient receives a $10,000 bill, they pay $10,000.

Somewhere along the line, the insurance company had assigned an outside doctor of their choice to oversee Andie's case. "Isn't that like the fox guarding the hen house?" Karen's husband Pete asked one night when I was picking up Tuck.

We quietly voiced our concerns about the potential conflict of interest to the nurses, but they assured us they wouldn't let Andie go home until she was ready. They also reiterated how much better babies thrive and grow once they're in their home environment. I assumed they were talking about babies with capable and confident mothers.

It wasn't until the day Tucker finally held his baby sister for the first time, nearly three months after her birth, that I started to understand where Andie really belonged. He sat in Lee's lap, wearing khaki pants and a white long-sleeved shirt with a hunter-green vest. His feet were crossed at the ankles. "I'm ready, Mama," he said. "I know, buddy," I said. "Marcia's getting her."

I held the camera ready as Marcia placed Andie on Tucker's lap. Through the camera lens, his apple cheeks were bursting with pride. Tears ran off Lee's chin onto Tuck's soft blond hair. I snapped photos and Marcia stood over my shoulder enticing Tucker with exclamations of "Cheeseburger!"

"Cheeseburgah!" he'd call back, smiling up at the camera.

I had tried to convince myself I really wanted Andie to come home, but at that moment, I began to feel like it might actually be true.

The next day, I looked down at Andie in her crib, trying to imagine her leaving the hospital and living with us. I just couldn't picture it. Then I thought of Tucker, waiting to be a real big brother, and I said out loud to anyone who was willing to listen, "I'm ready for her to come home."

That was me. I had said it. And I almost really meant it.

The next step before her discharge was to schedule the surgery to repair her iliostomy and remove that ostomy bag. We agreed it was best for her to have the surgery before she left the hospital, rather than readmit her after she'd been discharged. It was comforting to know she'd recover in her familiar NICU home with her own nurses caring for her.

The ostomy bag was a constant, glaring reminder of how close we'd come to losing her. It emerged just above her diaper and held a loop of intestine, where her poop came out. Because it never reached her bowel at the bottom of her intestine where water is absorbed, it was yellow, watery stool.

Marcia asked several times if we'd heard anything about a surgery date. We hadn't, so she offered to follow up with the surgeon and find out how soon the surgery could be scheduled. I wasn't that anxious about this surgery. I was looking forward to her growing belly being restored to the smooth, flat tummy it was meant to be. Now that Andie was bigger and healthier, I felt she would recover well, especially under the care of her nurses who'd nurtured her to health in the first place.

Or not.

Marcia received word from the surgeon that he would *not* perform the surgery before Andie went home. He claimed he'd said right from the beginning that the ostomy reversal wouldn't happen until Andie was at least a year old, or weighed ten kilos, whichever came first. I thought ten kilos couldn't be *that* much until Marcia told me it was twenty-two pounds. Andie hadn't even met the four-pound mark.

We'd done no more than *look* at Andie's ostomy bag. We had no idea how to properly care for it, let alone change it.

Just a week before, the prospect of Andie coming home was nearly impossible to comprehend, but I'd come around. Facing the scenario of bringing home an already vulnerable baby *with an ostomy bag* was too much. "I'm not a nurse," I said again, more desperately this time. Marcia patted my back. "Don't worry," she said.

Word spread among the nurses about the surgeon's insistence on waiting. Many of them stopped by Andie's station to express their annoyance, calling the doctor "old school" and saying that all the young surgeons were closing ostomies before the babies went home. "Contact another surgeon," they said, but we felt indebted to the one who had saved Andie's life. We called and begged him to perform the surgery before she went home, but he wouldn't budge. "One year or ten kilos," he insisted, and lectured us on the risks of performing the surgery when the intestines were still so small. "Why not wait?" he asked.

Why not wait? Where did I start? What if I told him the medical aspect of the bag wasn't my only worry? The fact was, it looked disgusting. I wanted Andie to be a pretty little baby with a rough start, who had all that behind her. I'd dress her in sweet little outfits and pretend we didn't even know what the NICU was. I wanted my baby to come home whole and beautiful. I felt like the doctor already knew that and just wanted me to say it out loud.

Lee and I talked again about contacting another surgeon, but we still felt reluctant to do so. Not only had this surgeon saved her life, but all the other surgeons were his colleagues. What if he was pissed off enough to tell his surgical buddy to screw up the surgery? Our biggest fear was that he was actually right: It was safer to hold off until Andie, and her intestines, were bigger.

We decided to wait. Thus began our crash course in Ostomy Care 101.

I agreed to learn proper ostomy care, but deep down I didn't really believe I needed it. I thought the surgeon would change his mind. Something would change. Something *had* to change. There was no way I'd be doing this for the next year.

With the bag removed, Andie's ostomy was wet and slimy, resembling a jumbo-sized pink thimble. It was shocking to see part of an intestine on the outside of the body. The nurses made it look easy, but I felt awkward and clumsy when faced with it.

"Okay." Marcia pushed her glasses up on her nose, "You ready to learn this?" When I said no, she laughed.

I picked up my pencil and wrote "#1" in my notebook as Marcia began the demonstration.

"The key to the ostomy bag is putting it on really good and hoping it stays attached for as many days as possible." I wrote this down. "Make sure you have all your supplies right next to you." I looked up. She pointed to the adhesive remover, skin protector, pencil, paste, measuring guide, gauze, alcohol wipes, plastic bags, new pouch, and scissors. I knew

I was in trouble. I could barely wrap a birthday present without taping my fingers together.

I went through five ostomy bags on my first try. Marcia watched over me. "That's okay," she said with each one I threw in the trash. "You'll get it." Andie lay patiently on the table as I fumbled with her intestine. The stoma was so slimy, every time I touched it my mind screamed, *Ick! You're touching the inside of your daughter's body.* I tried not to look disgusted, but it *was* disgusting.

First, I cut the adhesive portion of the bag, then I swabbed the skin around the ostomy with an alcohol wipe, and finally I squeezed a line of medical cement around the stoma and the opening of the bag. This had to be done quickly, because if any stool came out during the process, I had to start all over. The final step was to fit the cutout over the ostomy, squishing it together as it slid through the cut hole. Knowing firsthand how an intestine felt, especially that of your child, is something I never imagined I'd have to find out.

As I worked at learning it, I kept thinking of all the bridal shower and wedding gifts I'd tried to wrap. I always wound up swearing and throwing the tape across the room. Lee would step in and calmly wrap the gifts with his precise folds and well-tied bows. I thought maybe we could do the same with the ostomy bag. "Uh, there's a little problem with that plan," he said. "I'll be at work all day."

"That's okay," I said. "I'll wrap her in a towel and wait for you to get home."

By the time I knew how to somewhat successfully change an ostomy bag, it was mid-February and I wanted the whole

NICU experience over. I was done, ready to take my baby—ostomy and all—and get the hell out of there.

Just days away from Andie's discharge, my friend, Sandy, offered to drive up from Connecticut and take Tucker for two nights so we could get away. Sandy was practically part of our family. She'd been our babysitter since she was 14, and I was nine. My dad gave her away at her wedding, and she did a reading at ours. "Sandy, that's too much," I told her over the phone.

"But this is something I really want to do," she said.

"Are you sure?" I asked.

"Very sure," she said. "I cannot wait to get up there and get my hands on Tucker."

I pictured him curled up in Sandy's arms. At 14 she'd been taller than all the boys, rail thin with long, straight brown hair. As an adult, her hair had gone blond, and she was the gorgeous mom of two boys.

I said yes.

We traveled north for two days of skiing. In the mountains the smell of fresh snow mingled with wood smoke and made my skin tingle. Lee reached his hand across the seat to hold mine. It was the only skiing we'd get in that year. Once away, we realized just how much we needed time together. I kept saying it should be mandatory for couples to take a couple of days away together before their baby comes home.

On our first day away, we discussed all we'd been through, and everything that was to come.

On our second day, we hardly talked at all. We didn't need to. We just skied. At noon we sat together on an outdoor deck and drank beers. We were 21 again, young and free. Kids? What kids? Hospital? What hospital?

"Let's not go back," I said.

Lee didn't respond. He didn't need to.

✦

And then we *were* back, a little less tired and a little more hopeful. We were ready—ready for our future to begin, with Andie at home.

We carried the car seat in for the customary hospital check. The nurse said we would have to wrap a towel around her head because it was too small for the car seat. We packed a bin of her teeny preemie clothes. We practiced being "alone" with our baby in one of the family rooms off of the waiting room. We were as ready as we were ever going to be.

And then, once again, just as we had that golden ring nearly in our grasp, the carousel lurched, and we missed it.

Andie needed another surgery. This time, it was her eyes.

17

Cowgirls

✦

CERTAIN ANIMALS are fight animals while others are flight animals. A provoked or scared lion sets up to fight. A horse startles and takes flight. It's the same way with people. Some run away and others stay to look fear in the eye. Ever since Andie's birth I'd been galloping away like a skittish, young filly.

When we found out Andie needed another surgery, the tiny amount of juice left in my adrenals tried to rev me up. But there wasn't enough. I was too tired to fly and had no interest in a fight.

In a conference room off the NICU, we were introduced to Dr. V. Lee sat with his fists clenched and his jaw set, ready to take everyone on. I sat next to him with slumped shoulders, my mind swirling, thinking how I must have created this scenario by not wanting Andie to come home. Dr. V. looked about our age, thin, fair-skinned, and intelligent. "So here's the deal," she said, and off I went. I didn't have the fuel to flee, so I floated. My kite string unraveled, and up I rose. As words fell from her lips, I noticed her glasses, wondering if they were a prerequisite for an eye doctor. I gazed at the ceiling, trying to figure out why the lighting in the room felt different. I looked over at Lee who was listening intently. I wanted to be alone with him, curled up on our couch, watching a movie. I wanted the doctor to stop talking so Lee could tell me everything she said.

"You're going to do the surgery *today?*" Lee asked.

My kite string yanked hard, and I came toppling back to the ground.

"Yes, today."

I looked at my watch. It was just after six in the evening.

"That is, if you agree to enroll her in our research study and the computer pulls her name."

"Wait." I looked at Lee. "What?"

Lee glanced at the doctor and then leaned toward me. "They want to do the surgery now," he said quietly.

I looked at the doctor's prim hands, folded on the shiny wood table in front of her. "What surgery?" I asked. "What do you mean?"

Dr. V. took a deep breath.

"Weren't you listening?" Lee asked.

I slumped in my chair. "Sort of."

"Okay," Dr. V. drew the word out like it was three syllables. "Preemies are prone to retinopathy." She closed her eyes, as though exasperated she had to go through all this again. I felt Lee reach over and take my hand. Mine was limp in his. "A full-term baby is born with fully developed retinas, but preemie retinas are still forming." The doctor opened her eyes; they were the color of steel. "Retinopathy of prematurity, or ROP, happens when the development of the retina stops and then starts again." She quickly brushed a stray hair from her cheek. "The new growing blood vessels are often abnormal and cause scar tissue. The purpose of the laser surgery is to destroy the growth of these abnormally developing vessels. The early results from the research study will allow us to perform retinal surgery sooner than we originally thought." She looked from me to Lee and back again. "Typical surgical standards require retinopathy to progress to a stage three before surgery can be considered. The study was designed to prove that surgery performed in stage two, rather than waiting until stage three, will be more successful."

"Stage two?" I looked at Lee. "Stage three?"

"There's a sliding scale of severity ranging from one to five," Dr. V said. "One is the least acute case of retinopathy, five is a detached retina, or blindness."

My flight response finally kicked in. I wanted to run from stage five.

"If you'll agree to enroll her in the research study," Dr. V. started to say.

But before she could continue, I interrupted, "Yes we will. We want the surgery now. That's what we want."

Lee put his hand on my leg to settle me down.

Dr. V. cleared her throat. "Just so you understand," she said, "It's a blind study."

A *blind* study. I didn't point out her ridiculous choice of language.

"We'll only do the surgery early if the computer pulls her name. There's a fifty-fifty chance . . ."

It turned out I had more adrenal juice left than I thought. "Please just pick her name," I begged. I felt hysterical at the prospect of leaving Andie's fate up to a computer. "We agree to do the surgery *now*."

Dr. V. swallowed. "Deliberately choosing a patient's name would compromise the legitimacy of the study," she had a maddeningly level, professional voice.

"I don't care about legitimacy," I told her. "This is *our baby* at risk."

Dr. V. rose. "Let's see what happens," she said.

After she left the room, I realized I was shaking. Lee pulled me into his arms. I rattled into his chest about all the worthless lottery tickets I'd ever bought and the prizes I'd never won.

When the door finally opened, I looked up. Dr. V. had a smile on her face.

"Well," she said, sitting down in front of us again. "The computer chose Andie's name."

I can't remember exactly what I said, but it was probably something like, "Yes. Let's get this surgery started." But Lee had different thoughts. He was still in fight mode. "Why should you be the doctor who is going to perform this surgery?" I heard him say.

My cheeks burned. Grabbing his upper arm, I whispered. "Lee."

He shook off my hand, ignoring me. "Even the best doctors in the world have a bad day," he said. "How do I know this won't be one of yours?"

Dr. V. was a fight animal, too. She sat up taller in her chair and responded through a tight smile, citing her list of impressive credentials as if she were on a job interview, which I guess she kind of was. I half expected her to pull out a résumé.

Panicked and embarrassed, I desperately wanted to say, "Wow! What a list of qualifications!" But I sat stone silent. This wasn't my fight.

Lee leaned further forward, his eyes still locked on hers. "How many of these surgeries have you performed?" Dr. V. paused. I held my breath. Her eyes went up to the left side of the room, as though she were counting. After a long moment, she looked back. Shrugging, she said, simply, "Hundreds."

Good enough for me. Not for Lee.

"Are you sure you're alert enough at this time of night to perform this surgery?" I glanced at my watch again. It was now close to 7 P.M.

"I am." She spoke with unwavering certainty.

I waited.

Lee looked at the floor. Finally, he raised his eyes to hers. "Okay," he said.

◆

Andie was taken into a small operating room in the NICU, while we went to stare at the fish tank in the waiting room.

I was worried Lee had pissed off Dr. V. "What were you thinking?" I wanted to ask him. You can't speak to doctors that way. She holds our baby's future in her hands. Doctors should be revered and praised, then they like you and try their hardest to do the best job possible. But I saw the look in his eyes, and I said nothing. His intense, furious gaze scared me. I could feel the scream waiting in his throat.

Resigned to sit in silence, I watched the fish swim back

and forth in their tank, bumping up against the glass. Then I
remembered there was something I *could* do. Sitting back, I
closed my eyes and visualized that blue healing light traveling
down from above, directly into Andie's right eye.

An hour later, Dr. V. came into the waiting room, with a
paper mask hanging around her neck and her hair tucked under a surgical cap. "All set," she said. She brushed her palms
together. "She did really well. The surgery was a success."
Lee stood to shake her hand. I buried my face in my hands
and felt the hot tears come. "Thank you for taking care of our
daughter," I heard Lee say. Dr. V. told him he was welcome.
I lowered my hands from my face and watched her head toward the elevators.

A nurse took us back to see Andie. "Don't be alarmed,"
she said, "But we had to move her back into NICU B while
she recovers." NICU B was the room with the blaring alarms
and thick, terrified air that Andie had been in for so long
after she was born. Walking in that room was like going back
in time. "It's okay," the nurse said. "She'll be out of here by
morning."

But she wasn't. The next morning, the nurse met me at
the door to say Andie had struggled throughout the night and
wasn't coming out of the anesthesia well. They'd had to intubate her in the middle of the night. When I saw her asleep
with the breathing tube in her throat, fear and panic rose up
in me. Her face was ashen, her eyes were squeezed shut, and
the breathing tube contorted her lips. It might have been
my imagination, but I thought the nurses wouldn't meet my
gaze. I called Lee from the waiting room and poured my

panic through the phone line. He raced over in a cab. We stood looking down at Andie's isolette. "Please get better," I begged her. "You've come too far to leave now." We stood in silence for a long time until Lee said, "We want you to come home now, Andie."

She began improving later that the day. By late evening, she was off oxygen and moved back into the intermediate NICU.

Someone once told me you had to fall off a horse three times before you could be considered a cowgirl. Three surgeries later, I'd say Andie was one hell of a cowgirl.

18

Family

⁂

DOROTHY KNOWS there's no place like home. We'd
walked the yellow brick road; met the Scarecrow, the
Tin Man, and the Cowardly Lion along the way. We'd found
our brains, heart, and courage and just had to put Andie in
those ruby red slippers, click her heels, and bring her home.
But before we could do that, we had to spend a morning in
the NICU practicing being alone with her.

As Yvonne wheeled the plastic crib slowly toward the
family room, Tucker reached his pudgy hand up to help her.
Lee and I followed behind. Passing nurses smiled and offered
congratulations. "You made it," they said.

The family room was decorated with an office-style
couch, two chairs, and a TV. Yvonne stood in the doorway.
"Relax and enjoy your time together." We nodded and sat on
the edge of the couch in front of the crib. "I'm sure gonna
miss her." Yvonne's voice cracked as she looked at the crib.
"You just come to love 'em so much." And then her fairy-like
body glided back out of the room.

Lee picked up Andie and sat with her in a corner of the
couch. Tucker quickly climbed up next to him and put his
fingers on her cheeks. Her mouth formed a little "O" shape,
and we laughed as she turned her face to grab his fingers.

And then we all just sat there. Lee and I looked at each other wishing we knew what to do.

"How long do we stay?" Lee asked.

I shook my head. "I don't know. How about a video?"

Tuck jumped off the couch in excitement. The choices were limited, so we picked a *Barney* video over *The Wiggles*.

Tucker cuddled in next to Lee, who slid further down on the couch. Soon Andie was fast asleep, facedown on his chest, just like Tucker had done so many times when he was a baby. Lee closed his eyes and Tucker held onto Andie's fingers. I sat studying my little brood as the dinosaur sang, "I love you, you love me, we're a happy fam-i-ly." Lee opened one eye and gave me a big satisfied smile. I giggled, let out a breath, and rested back on the couch.

The next morning, I lay in bed, staring up at the freshly painted ceiling. Somehow Lee had done it; he'd managed to get our bedroom finished in time. We'd had to cut some corners, we'd wanted wide pine floors like the rest of the house, but a guy from the local home store installed wall-to-wall carpeting over the plywood subfloor. "I love it," I'd assured Lee. "It's so cozy." We also hadn't had time to paint it ourselves, so we hired a friend's painting crew to cover our bedroom walls in the green paint I'd seen at a friend's house. "Camouflage," she told me when I called for the paint color. "It changes color depending on the light, from green to gray to blue."

One of the painters was tall with soft brown skin and gorgeous green eyes. "I feel sorry about your baby," he said to me. My friend who owned the company later told me the painter's three-year-old daughter had fallen out a second story window. "Her initial tests look okay," my friend said, "But they don't know what it means for the long term."

I looked at the white wicker bassinet at the end of our sleigh bed and the stack of preemie books on my bedside table. I wondered what the long term meant for us.

Lee's leg was draped over mine, and his breath tickled my neck. "Whatcha thinking?" he asked.

"I thought you were asleep."

"You're obviously not. What's up?"

"What's up?" I asked. "Are you joking?"

"You ready?"

"I don't know," I brought the blanket up to my chin. "It's hard to believe she's actually coming home." He pulled his leg off and wrapped his fingers in mine. "It's time, Kase. She needs to be here with us." He propped himself on his elbow and looked down at me. His eyes glowed green in the morning light from the window. I tried to bury my face in his faded t-shirt, but he took my chin between his fingers and lifted my face to his. "Hey, you're a good mom," he said. "You're gonna do great." He ran his hand through my hair. "Say you believe me."

I looked at the photo of Tucker on the mirror above my dresser, beaming as he held Andie in his lap. "I believe you," I said, but even I could hear doubt in my voice.

Fifteen minutes later, I stood on the soft green carpet in our new bedroom closet, wondering why I had all these clothes and what I was supposed to wear on bring-your-daughter-home-from-the-NICU day. I wanted to dress up, but it was late February, and my snow boots would look ridiculous with a skirt. We had enough going on without carrying along an extra pair of shoes just for the hospital. I ripped the tags off a new white blouse. With black stretch pants, I'd look half dressed up.

After I got dressed, I stood looking at myself in the full-length mirror. I'd lost weight, and had dark circles under my eyes.

"We should get moving, babe." Lee called from downstairs. "Charlotte will be here any minute." I could hear *Sesame Street* playing on the kitchen TV below. My friend, Charlotte, was on her way to watch Tuck. A stack of white diapers and ostomy supplies waited next to Andie's changing table. I'd lined up cans of formula on the kitchen counter downstairs. Luckily, it was the weekend and Lee would be home. What was I going to do when I was alone with the kids? I couldn't imagine.

Driving in, Lee had his game face on. I sat in the passenger seat with my water, Brain Gym exercises, and a bottle of Rescue Remedy, the calming homeopathic flower mixture I'd learned about from Karen McCarthy, who had helped us prepare for Andie's upcoming discharge and our expectations of life at home.

Fortunately, Andie weighed over four pounds now and was coming home toward the beginning of spring, rather than the illness-infused winter season. Still, she was really vulnerable. Because her lung tissue was still regenerating and her immune system was still fragile, we couldn't have a big celebratory homecoming, and visitors would have to be kept to a minimum. We'd also have to avoid taking her to public places like drugstores, grocery stores, the library, and Tuck's school. Tucker and the germs he brought home from preschool would be her biggest health threat. Any illness could set her back and put her in the hospital again.

When Lee turned the car into the hospital parking garage, my stomach was in knots.

"We're here," he said.

"No shit," I said. I stretched my limbs in every direction and let out a big nervous scream.

Mingled with trepidation, and the sorrow of having to say goodbye to the nurses we loved because they'd loved Andie, I also felt the bittersweet excitement of finally bringing our baby home, and the relief of no longer making the daily trip into the hospital.

Like a graduating senior, I walked slowly into the NICU, trying to capture and remember everything familiar. I pointed out all our "last times"; *last time pushing number six in the elevator, last time walking past the collages of NICU graduates in the hallway, last time checking in with Zelda, last time washing our hands at the sink* . . . until Lee finally rolled his eyes and said, "Enough."

Marcia was waiting at Andie's station. Around her crib, the walls and shelves were bare. All her homemade get-well signs and family photos had been packed up, and a small plastic tub had been filled with a few preemie outfits and diapers. "She's been waiting for you," Marcia said. Looking at her familiar face, I felt the hot sting of tears. "Oh, don't start that yet," she said. "We still have some things to do here." I walked over and hugged her anyway. She patted my back. "Tina and Janice said goodbye to her last night, but they asked me to send their goodbyes along to you, too."

"Come home with us, Marcia," I said.

"I'd love to, but I know at some point my husband and kids would notice I was missing." She put her arm around me. "Besides, you're gonna be great."

We sat in the glider by Andie's crib and Marcia opened a large, three-ring binder on her lap. She went over the recipe for Andie's high-calorie formula and told us the dates of follow-up doctor's appointments. Then she carefully pushed the papers back over the rings and closed the binder. "Well, I think that's it," she said. "Unless you have any other questions." I raised my eyebrows. "No, I won't move in with you," she said.

"You know her too well," Lee said. We all laughed, even as the tears were sliding down our cheeks.

Then I snapped photos of Marcia with Andie, and Lee with Marcia and Andie. Lee snapped a few of me with Marcia and Andie. As he strapped Andie into the car seat to take her outside, I snapped pictures of her station, the room, and the view outside the window. "Okay, babe," Lee said. "That's enough. We should get going."

Lee carried Andie in her car seat, and Marcia walked with her arm around me. We waited at the bank of elevators that would lead us to the exit. My fingers lightly touched the corners on the metal frame of a NICU graduate's collage. "She'll be up there someday," Marcia said. I looked at an empty space on the wall where Andie's collage would fit.

Lee pressed the down button. As we waited for the elevator to arrive, we hugged Marcia one last time. "We'll come and visit," I said.

"You just stay home where you belong and enjoy your family," she said. We heard a ding and the metal doors slid open. Lee picked up Andie in her car seat and we leaned forward, but we didn't step in. "You can do this," Marcia said from behind us. "You're going to be great."

And then we both took that step forward into the elevator. "Thank you for everything," one of us said, and as the elevator doors closed, Marcia disappeared from view, and we both burst into tears.

19

Scars

✦

ANDIE ARRIVED HOME on February 23, 2001, weighing four pounds, fourteen ounces. She had spent 84 days in the hospital.

I sat in the back behind Lee, holding fast to her car seat, looking out at the snow-patched yard. Someone had hung balloons from the porch rail. Twisting in the wind, the mylar proclaimed, "It's a girl."

No kidding, I thought, but I kept my comment to myself. The sun was straining through a cover of steel-colored clouds. We were home, and I was supposed to be happy. Never mind that her poop collected in a bag attached to her abdomen, never mind that she'd just started taking bottles a few weeks ago, and that while she was eating there were still times she stopped breathing and needed to be startled back to life. Never mind that everything about this baby terrified me. Never mind all that, because we were home.

Lee turned the car off. "You ready?" he asked.

I nodded. "Ready as I'll ever be."

✦

I followed him through the back door as he carried Andie's car seat into the house and set her on the table. It was dark and quiet in the kitchen. I reached for the light, but pulled my hand off the switch when I saw Tucker and Charlotte standing in the doorway. Tucker walked over, looking shy and uncertain. "You want to help me get her out of here, big guy?" Lee pointed to Andie, asleep in the car seat. Tucker nodded. As Lee unbuckled her, I watched Charlotte pick up her coat and walked toward the door. "You don't have to go," I said. She glanced at Tucker, helping Lee lift Andie out of her car seat. "It's so good she's home, Kase." She took my hand; it was warm and solid in mine. "Yeah," I said, "It is." I hugged her and then watched her walk out the back door, her back hunched against the cold.

Leaning against the door, I let out a big breath. Lee sat on a kitchen chair with Andie in his arms. Tuck perched on his knee and peered into Andie's face. "Your sister's home," Lee whispered. I could tell he was holding back tears.

"Hey, Tuck," I said. "Andie brought you a present from the hospital." He looked up expectantly as I reached into the canvas bag at my feet.

"What did your sister bring you?" Lee asked.

I held the unwrapped gift behind my back. "Ready big guy?" Tucker closed his eyes and held out his hands. I put the binoculars down in his chubby palms. "Okay," I said.

His eyes popped open. "Binoculars!" he leaned close to her face. "Thanks Andie!"

We watched him put the plastic strap around his neck and hold the binoculars to his eyes. "Other way," Lee said, turning them around. Tucker turned around the room, looking at everything until he finally trained the binoculars on his sister. "She's bigger," he said.

And suddenly, I recognized the irony of the present.

We'd given him a gift whose only purpose was to make things appear larger.

✦

Later that night, I watched Andie sleeping in the wicker bassinet that Tucker's doll had slept in before she came home. I studied the little scar above her upper lip. It was from the tape that had held the breathing tube in place for so long. I wondered if it would ever go away. There were other little scars on her ankles and wrists from the tubes, needles, and tape. And there were scars from her surgeries: one across the right side of her belly, another jagged one under her left shoulder blade.

I brushed my fingers lightly across her cheek. I thought about how scared we'd been, walking through the hospital doors earlier that afternoon. Scared and scarred. Andie's scars were physical; the human eye could easily see them. No one could see our scars, but they were still there, deep and real and painful.

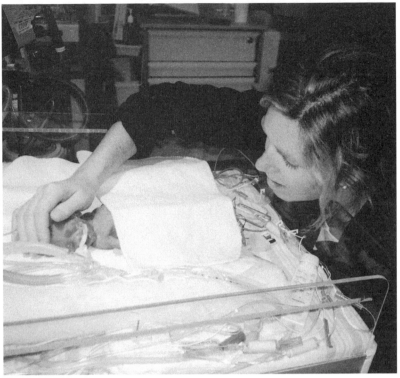

PHOTO: ELIZABETH ORMISTON

Could this really be my baby?

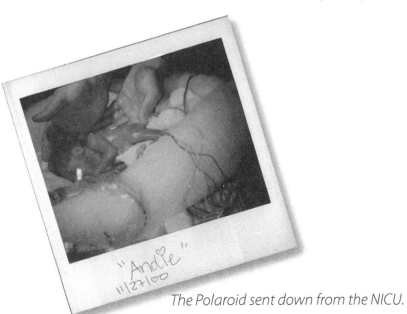

"Andie ♡"
11/27/00

The Polaroid sent down from the NICU.

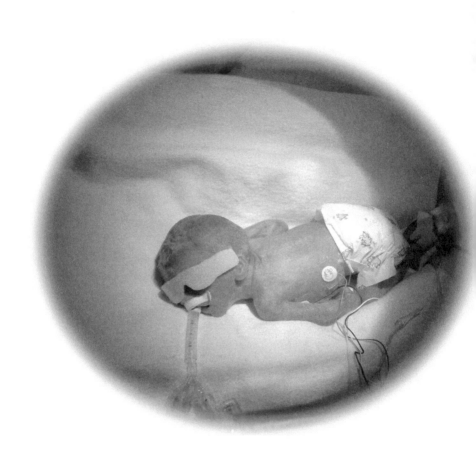

Andie,
1 pound, 11 ounces;
11 inches long.

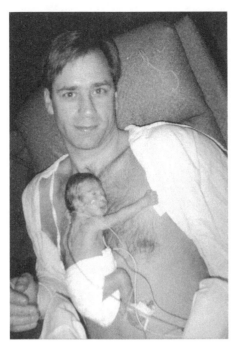

Lee came straight from work for a chance at Kangaroo care.

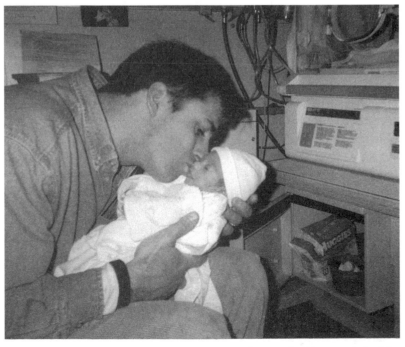

Lee—the devoted daddy.

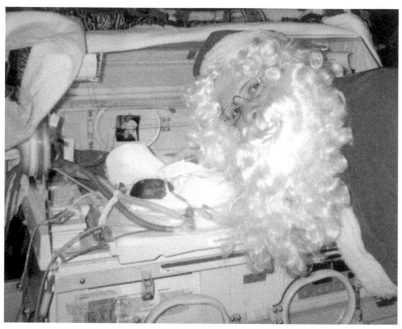

Andie's visit with Santa!

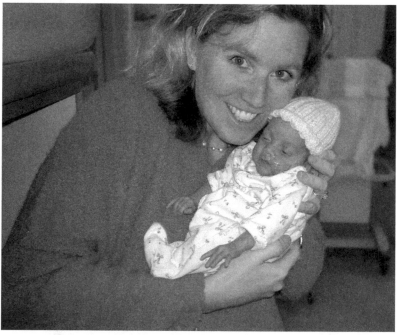

There's a lot of fear hiding behind that smile.

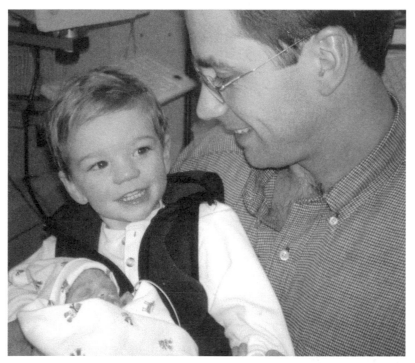

Tucker's first time holding his baby sister.

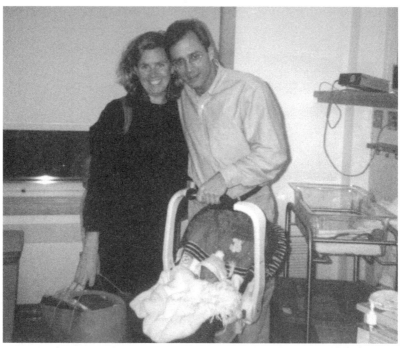

The big day taking Andie home—we're excited and terrified!

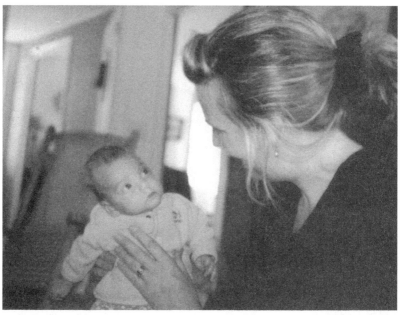

Finally at home, getting to know each other.

Ordinary days.

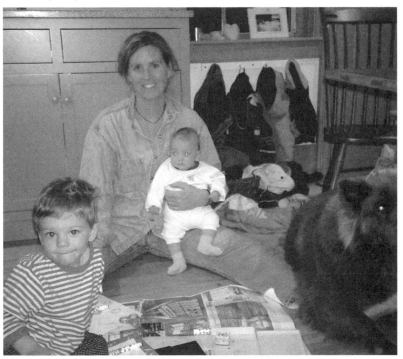

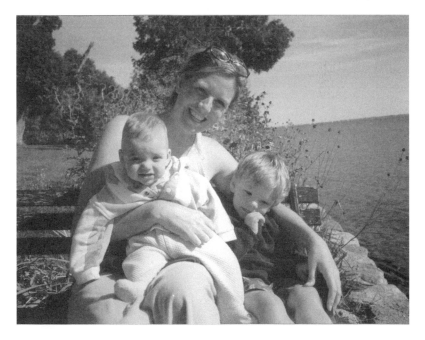

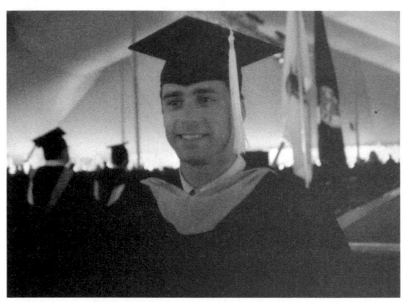

I don't know how Lee did it!

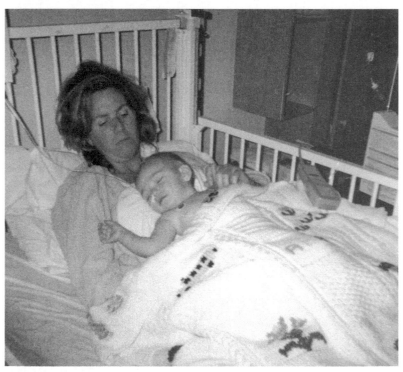

Recovering from ostomy-reversal surgery.

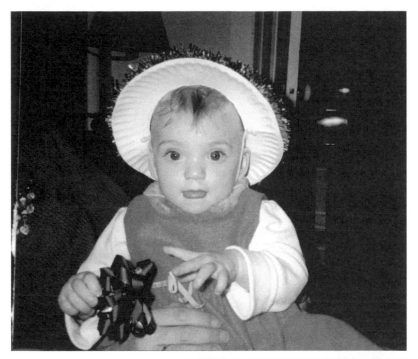

Andie's first Christmas at home.

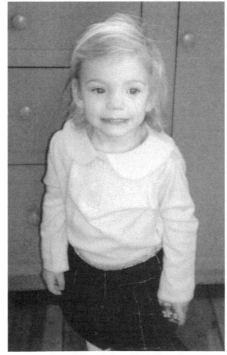

Andie's 2nd birthday. We thought we were safe.

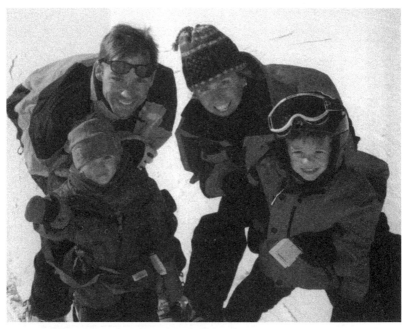

Andie's first time on skis, two years old.

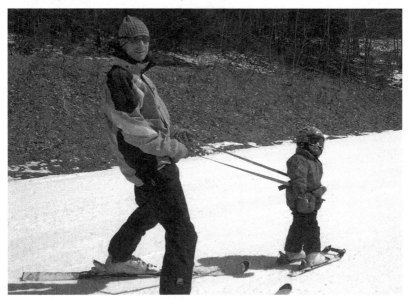

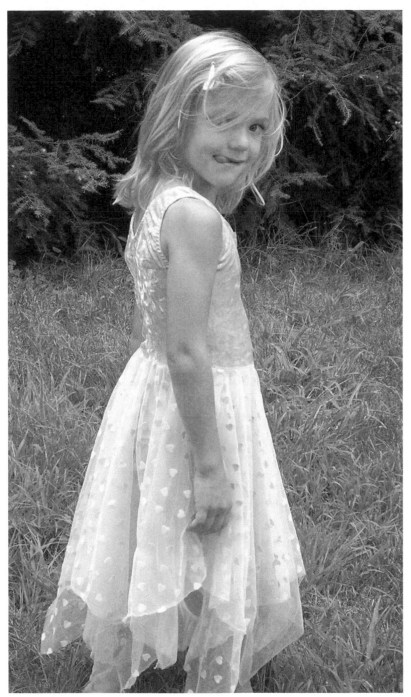

My 5-year-old vision realized.

Everyone gathered for Andie's baptism.

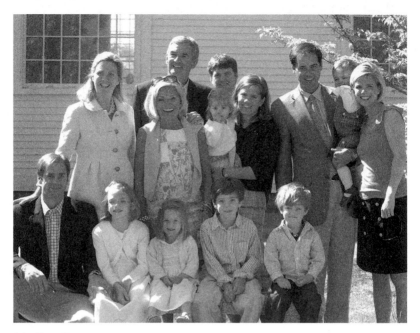

My family.

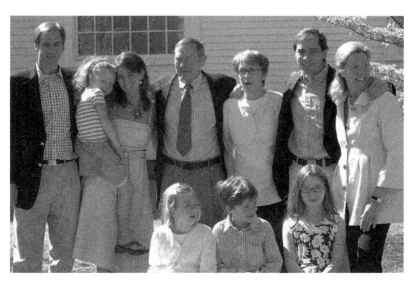

Lee's family.

Brotherly love.

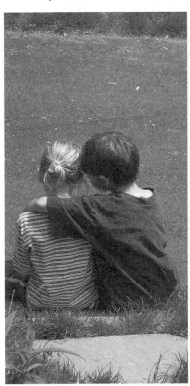

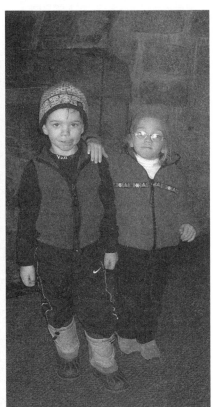

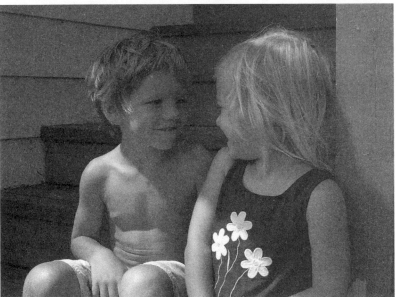

There's nothing Andie won't try!

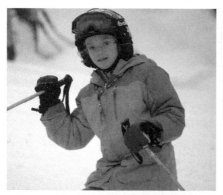

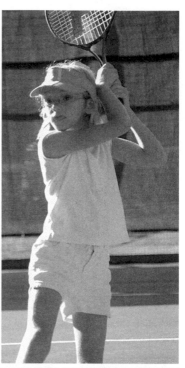

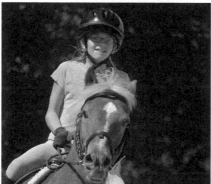

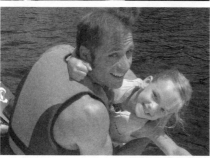

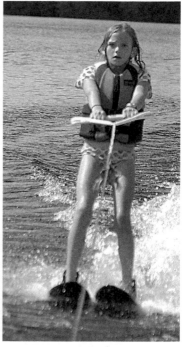

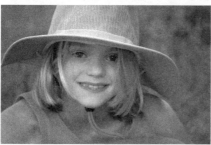

Part II

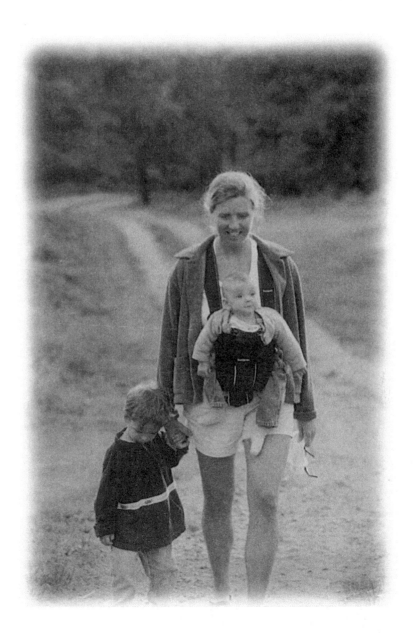

20

Crystal Ball

✦

R ACING BACK AND FORTH from the hospital had been
so intense. It was such a daily rush that on the morning
it suddenly ceased, and I went from 60 to 0, I wasn't sure
what to do. I was the mother of two young children living
under one roof, just what I'd been hoping for, and though I
was relieved, I was also terrified. There was no running from
the reality of my life—it was staring back at me through the
eyes of my two young children.

I imagined I was on a movie set. A director yelled cut
and someone shouted, "Andie's birth—take two."

Part of the terror was that I didn't know what to expect.
Thank God I couldn't see the future. If I'd had a crystal ball
that morning, it would have told me that every day I would
feel tentative, full of uncertainty. I'd cry often. Watching
television programs about healthy babies, I'd sob until I had
no tears left. I'd spend hours hovering over Andie as she slept
in that white bassinet, making sure she was still breathing.
Though there would be constant phone calls and packages
filled with pink onesies, soft receiving blankets, and picture
books, I would have the constant, dull ache of loneliness in
my belly.

Outside Tucker's preschool, I would try to make myself
take him inside while clutching Andie in my arms and imag-

ining all the germs waiting to snatch her from me. Finally, I'd have to ask another parent to take him in.

On Monday, Wednesday, and Friday mornings I'd bring Andie home, wishing Tuck was there to erase the silence in the house. Spreading towels out on the kitchen counter, I'd lay her down several times each day and empty her ostomy bag, gagging as liquid poop dripped off my fingers into the sink. I'd leave her sitting in her vibrating bouncy seat more than I should.

Teams of early intervention specialists—occupational therapists, physical therapists, and speech therapists—would walk through my front door. Reading the physical therapist's report, I'd smile when it said Tucker, with his ability to engage and challenge Andie, was by far her best therapist. I'd file the reports in a manila folder marked "Andie" with a little heart drawn over the "i."

In the grocery store, I'd watch new moms accept praise and smiles from passing shoppers and pretend I didn't care that my baby was too susceptible to illness to come grocery shopping.

I would feel lonely.

I'd complain to my family about the unending stream of doctor's appointments and standing in hospital elevators, I'd tell strangers (whether they cared to know or not) that the child in my arms had been born four months prematurely. I'd smile when they said she was a miracle. I'd see other parents pushing their children in wheelchairs and want to tell them, *I know, I get it, I'm in that club.* But I'd look away, feeling guilty, believing my own child would walk someday.

Every time I drove that same road leading to the hospital, even if only for a routine visit, my old anxieties and fears would return, along with recurring bouts of diarrhea, forcing me to learn which coffee shops had public restrooms.

When Lee passed through the back door each night, I'd run into his arms. As he tenderly kissed each of his children, I would see pure, genuine love radiating from him and wish he was the one who stayed home with them.

If I'd had that crystal ball I would have seen myself looking into the mirror above the bathroom sink, staring into the eyes of a frightened woman I no longer knew and wondering what the rest of her life would bring.

2 1

Belief

✦

ONE LATE FEBRUARY EVENING, we bundled Andie in a warm fleece, left Tuck with a neighbor, and drove through the snowy streets to see Karen McCarthy.

Karen greeted us at the door with hugs. "Finally, the famous Andie," she said, pulling the blanket back from the car seat to get a better look. She put her hand on her heart. "She's beautiful." Lee and I smiled.

In her office, Lee set Andie down in her car seat in the corner, and we settled into our seats. Karen sat in her chair, looking at us with a strange smile on her face. We looked back, waiting for her to start the appointment. She kept staring. Nervously, I cleared my throat.

"What are you doing?" she asked.

Lee and I looked at each other. "What do you mean?" I asked.

She nodded at Andie. From her car seat in the furthest corner of the room, she was looking out at us with big eyes, her little nose poking out from under the hat and blanket she was still bundled in.

"What are you doing?" Karen asked again.

We'd been in Karen's office several times and she usually approached us, me in particular, with careful kindness. I didn't know where this new version of her was coming from, but I didn't like it. Folding my arms across my chest, I asked again, "What do you mean?"

"You two are sitting there, and your baby is all the way over there." Karen nodded again to Andie. "What's up with that?"

Neither of us moved or answered. I wanted to kick Lee in the ankle, and tell him to go pick Andie up, but we were both caught in Karen's headlights, too exposed to move. Lee's jaw was set in a tight line. I wiped my sweaty palms on the legs of my jeans.

Finally, Karen began again. "I just want to know why that baby isn't in your arms." She leaned forward, her long brown hair falling over her shoulders. "That baby has come into this world for a reason," she said. "She has a purpose. She's here to love you and be loved by you, and she worked long and hard to get here. She doesn't deserve to be shoved in a corner. She needs you, and she needs your love."

Neither of us moved. I mumbled something about her being happiest in her car seat.

Then Karen said what Lee and I had been thinking ever since Andie was born and what we would never say aloud. She said, "Andie is not going to die."

A sob escaped from deep inside me. Lee stood up, walked across the room, unbuckled Andie, and returned to his seat with her cradled in his arms. She gazed up at him from the crook of his elbow. "She's not going anywhere," Karen said with more softness in her voice.

I reached out and touched Andie's little fingers. "I'm so afraid."

"I know," Karen nodded, "But you're so afraid she'll die;

you're caring for her but you've closed yourselves off from loving her, really deeply loving her."

Karen reached over to her desk and passed me a box of tissues. "She is here to live. To live and be loved. You need to love her."

And there it was. The truth. The truth had finally been spoken out loud. There was nothing left for us to say. Karen had said it all.

✦

A few days later, we took Andie to the pediatrician; her first doctor's appointment away from the hospital. After the pediatrician examined her, he leaned against the counter, scribbling in her chart. He was wearing a cashmere V-neck sweater, and I noticed, while standing next to Lee and holding Andie in my arms, that his fingernails were manicured. "She'll always be small." He tapped his silver, engraved pen on the edge of his clipboard and glanced at Andie. "And, she'll have learning disabilities." He adjusted the trendy glasses that matched his sweater and began to brag about his ability to identify a preemie. I looked at the framed photos of his beautiful children hanging on the wall, while he told us about a Saturday on the soccer field when he picked a thin, young boy out of all the players on the turf. "I leaned into my wife," he said, "and told her, *that boy's a preemie.*" His wife knew the boy and told him he was right. "I can always tell," he said.

I looked him directly in the eye. "No," I said.

He took his glasses off. "No, what?"

I noticed for the first time the fine acne scars deeply imbedded in his cheeks.

"No, she won't be small." I said. "No, she won't have learning disabilities, and no, you will not be able to pick her out as a preemie."

He laughed. I guess he thought his medical degree entitled him to do so. We didn't laugh with him. Then he muttered something about my "state of denial" and looked at Lee, as though for backup.

Lee smoothed things over because he's good at that. "We're just trying to keep a positive attitude," he said.

But Lee and I both knew it wasn't just about attitude. It was about belief. It was about certainty. It was about knowing that our daughter came here to prove she would be so much more than anyone could ever imagine.

22

Buildings

◆

HENDERSON HARBOR is on the eastern edge of Lake Ontario an hour north of my parent's home. As a child, my grandmother vacationed there. Then she grew up and had children, and my mother and her two sisters vacationed there. And when my mother grew up and had children, my siblings and I vacationed there, too. My aunt and uncle still spend summers there, in the old turn-of-the-century ginger-bread cottages overlooking the harbor.

This was the spot I wrote about in English class when asked to close my eyes, picture my favorite place, and write in detail. I'd describe the wooden swing hanging from the old cedar tree, the long dirt road I meandered with a pack of water-logged dogs, the Queen Anne's lace and wild sweet pea dotting the fields. I'd write about the scent of bacon drifting from my grandmother's cottage, the sound of waves hitting the shore and how young, safe, and protected I felt.

There wasn't a summer in my life when I'd missed a visit to Henderson. But that first summer Andie was home, we decided not to go. We told each other the long, six-hour drive, the dusty old cottages, and the attention of all those wonderful relatives would just be too much. We needed quiet. We needed time just as a foursome. We needed to know ourselves as a family.

So we went to Cape Cod, a safe hour and a half from home. The cottage we rented was charming, a gray-shingled windmill in a boatyard just a short stroll to the beach and town center. Our time there was casual and unhurried, and we spent it sitting on the sand, playing in the yard, and standing under the spray of the outdoor shower. An easy baby with big, alert eyes and Lee's long lashes, Andie was getting rounder and cuter by the day. We spread a quilt out in the yard so she could lie down on it, and Tucker would blow strawberries on her belly. She'd howl laughing, grabbing fistfuls of his hair in her pudgy hands. He didn't seem to notice her ostomy bag, and during those leisurely times, we seemed to resemble a normal, vacationing family.

But an unwanted guest had refused to stay home—our old friend Fear had tagged along. At night, while lying in bed and watching the wooden blades of the windmill turn past the open window, our worries would return with the reminder that Andie's surgery still lay ahead. In an effort to enjoy the remainder of our respite, we sucked in our breath and tried to calm our edgy nerves.

The fear wasn't just about the surgery; it was about not knowing *when* the surgery would be. Andie's primary-care doctor warned us that scheduling a surgery too late in the fall could expose her to serious illness. "She could end up sharing a room with a child with RSV (Respiratory Syncytial Virus) or meningitis," he'd said. But fall was fast approaching, and the surgeon still refused to set a surgery date. An electric charge of anxiety churned just below the surface of our sun-tanned skin.

One morning about three or four days into our trip,

I was grabbing some towels from the line while Lee played kickball with Tucker, when a blond woman waved to me from the doorway of the next-door cottage. "Hey neighbor," she said. Her husband came up behind her and Lee and I walked over. We met by the split-rail fence that lined the property and exchanged the usual pleasantries; where we lived, jobs, colleges, and then *the question*—the one that caused our conversations to falter, "How old are your kids?"

Since Andie had come home, we'd been calculating her "real age" versus "corrected age." It drove me crazy. I'd barely passed Intro Math in college, or "potato- head math" as we called it. When Tucker was born I'd struggled to understand baby-age speak when other mothers said, "He's eighteen weeks tomorrow," or "Yesterday she was three and a half months." *How did someone know that?* I wondered and always answered: "Oh he's a few months old," "Around six months," or "Close to a year."

So calculating Andie's age based on her birthdate, November 27th, and then recalculating her age based on her due date, March 12th, was frustrating and confusing. I wondered how long we were going to go around spouting two ages for one child?

"Tucker's almost three," I said, then passed the baton to Lee.

"Well," he began. "Andie was born in November, but she was due . . ." *Blah, blah, blah,* "so now she's nine months old, or five months corrected."

The woman, her name was Kerry or Kathy, said "Twenty-five weeks?" She looked over at Andie, who was lying across her quilt on the lawn, gumming a ring toy and happily kicking her legs in the air. "*She* was born 25 weeks?"

She looked at her husband who raised his eyebrows.

"Yeah," Lee said, "Twenty-five weeks," like *You got a problem with that?*

"Oh my God," Kerry (or Kathy) said. "My sister just gave birth to a 25-weeker a month ago."

"You're kidding?" I stepped closer.

She went on to tell us everything about her niece's birth. When she was finished, I told them Andie's story.

They looked over at her again. "Wow, she looks so good."

How could it be that we wound up staying right next door to a family with our shared experience? Just a coincidence? No way. It had to be another of the many events orchestrated by some higher power.

At the end of the vacation we hugged our new friends, swapped addresses, and for a few years we exchanged Christmas cards.

✦

Back at home, I felt more rested and confident than I had in a long time. I also felt antsy and unsettled. I wanted to get away again, to keep moving.

After two days at home, I was loading the dishwasher when I picked up the phone and called Lee at work. He answered on the second ring. "I'm taking the kids to Henderson Harbor," I said.

"By yourself?"

"Yeah. I don't want to miss a summer there after all."

I kept loading dirty cereal bowls and sippy cups into the dishwasher while Lee voiced his concerns.

"Lee," I said. "How many times have I made that drive? I could do it with my eyes closed. Plus my whole family's gonna be there. It'll be great."

"Would you please stop clanging the dishes and sit down for a minute?"

I pulled a bar stool out from the kitchen island. "Okay, I'm sitting," I said, and he kept talking, but I wasn't really listening. I'd already started packing in my mind.

"I don't know," he said just before we hung up. "I don't feel right about this."

But I went to pull the dirty laundry out of the duffle bags that we hadn't even unpacked from the Cape.

I left the next morning. It was a long, tiring drive, and to keep myself going I imagined the big reception we'd receive once we arrived.

But when we drove down the steep, gravel driveway, the cottages looked empty and lonely, and no one came out to greet us. My grandparents were quietly puttering in their own world and didn't even hear us pull up. When I finally poked my head in to say hello, they said my Aunt Harriet and cousin Marnie were off looking at colleges, and Uncle Jeff was at work. My parents had just called to say they couldn't come up for a couple days.

Compared to the freedom of the beach where Tucker ran and dug in the sand, the lake was restrictive and dangerous. I kept screaming at him to stay away from the steep steps and the ten-foot stonewall that separated the lawn from the water. Andie had just started putting everything in her mouth and I was afraid to put her down. The cottage had old painted floors and ancient mothballs hidden in various corners.

Uh oh, I thought. But when I talked to Lee I told him everything was great.

"I'm so glad you got to go up there after all," he said.

"Oh yeah." I looked at a piece of broken wire jutting out from the screen door. "I can't believe I was going to miss this."

"You're sure you're okay there by yourself with the kids?"

"Oh yeah, this is great," I said.

But for two days I lived in constant fear that Tucker would fall off the stonewall or Andie would ingest something horribly poisonous. All the reserves I'd built up on the Cape leaked out, and the frayed edges I'd become so accustomed to had reemerged. I missed the comforts and ease of home. I craved our clean, carpeted rooms filled with age-appropriate toys and a VCR that played *Boys Love Trucks* videos.

Fortunately, my aunt and uncle returned and my parents were coming up the next day. Right after putting the kids down that second night, I collapsed into bed. As I reached up to pull the brass chain to switch off the light, I told myself that tomorrow would be better.

At midnight, I startled awake. My left arm was completely numb and the left side of my chest was burning in pain. I got out of bed, holding the wooden headboard with my right hand and trying to shake feeling back into my left arm. The numbness lingered. My chest was on fire. I couldn't take in a full breath. I walked out into the dark living room and dialed our home number on the old rotary phone. The phone rang and rang. The black receiver was heavy in my hand. I cursed our dial-up modem. Lee had gone to bed with the computer on again, tying up the phone line so I couldn't get through.

The lights were all out next-door. Sitting alone in the dark on the wooden arm of an old wing chair, I shook my arm, willing it back to life. "Damn it." I looked down at my watch. 12:30 A.M. I called my parents.

"Hello?" My dad's voice had the urgency of someone who'd been woken in the middle of the night.

"Dad?" I said.

"What's wrong?" he asked.

I tried to sound as casual as possible. "My arm is sort of numb and my chest hurts."

"*Your arm is numb and your chest hurts?*" he repeated. I heard fumbling over the phone line and my mother say, in her raspy half-asleep voice, "Give me the phone, Jerry," and then she was on the line. "Kasey, go next door right now and wake up Harriet and Jeff. You need to get to the hospital."

She knew 911 wasn't an option. We'd learned the hard way many years ago when my cousin Andrew rolled off the lawn and fell ten feet to the rocks below. Aunt Harriet rocked him in her arms, while the open gash on his forehead bled. "Where is that ambulance?" she kept asking. They eventually drove to the hospital. The ambulance couldn't get down the long, narrow harbor road.

"Kasey, put the phone down and go next door," Mom said.

In my bare feet, I padded across the dew-covered lawn, the pant legs of my pajamas brushing the wet grass and sticking to my calves. I opened the screen door as quietly as I could and stood in the silence of the living room, making one last attempt to erase the pain and numbness, but there was no use. I heard a snore come from upstairs and creeping up the wooden staircase, I quietly called out my aunt and uncle's names, "Harriet? Jeff?" The snoring continued. I stood just outside the open door of their bedroom, and said their names again, louder this time. "Harriet? Jeff?" Nothing.

Finally, I walked into their room and stood at the end of their bed. I was like a ghost, haunting them. I said their names again, touching my aunt's ankle, which was poking out from under the white comforter. They both startled and sat up, looking confused and concerned. "Mom and Dad told me to come get you," I said. "My arm is kind of numb and my chest hurts."

We'd had nighttime emergencies before, but they usually involved boats and storms. Still they were seasoned enough to snap into emergency mode. While my aunt tucked her nightgown into her jeans, she ordered my uncle next door to stay with my sleeping kids. Grabbing her car keys, she ushered me toward the car while I mumbled embarrassed apologies.

We drove to the closest hospital, about 35 minutes away. On the road there, we passed darkened farms and scattered homes. I imagined families sleeping soundly inside. I thought of Lee, sleeping alone in our bed, not knowing this was happening. I wanted to hear him tell me I was going to be okay.

I worried about the children waking up and finding their mommy gone.

The emergency room of the Watertown hospital was a striking contrast to the quiet, dark stillness of the outside world. Bright, fluorescent lights illuminated two families stationed in the waiting room. Both fathers wore camouflage green fatigues, declaring their affiliation with the local army base. The families stared at me and listened as I whispered my symptoms to the registering nurse. She looked bored and annoyed until I said chest pain, then her droopy, lifeless eyes widened. "Follow me." She led me back to a little cubicle and stuck my index finger in a clip attached to a small box. "To test your oxygen levels," she said. *Yeah, I know,* I thought. *My daughter had one taped to her foot for two months.* She handed me a thin hospital gown and began hooking up other monitoring devices, working quickly and concisely. There was no warmth in her actions.

Aunt Harriet came in after parking the car and pulled a chair up to the bed. Soon, a young doctor entered the tiny room. I could almost hear my aunt thinking, *Are you kidding me? This guy's not old enough to babysit my dog.* I shot her a look, and she hid a smirk behind her hand. The doctor began his exam, listening to my chest and checking my reflexes. When he finished, he stood at the end of the bed and looked down at a metal clipboard. He studied the page, flipped to the next, and then looked up. "I can't find anything wrong with you," he said.

"Nothing?" I asked. After waking everybody up and making such a scene, it had to be something. "Are you sure?"

"Pretty sure," he said. He looked back at the clipboard. "But even so, you should see your primary doctor tomorrow, especially if the pain and numbness don't go away."

I didn't say anything. He tapped his fingers on the clipboard. "Okay then." He nodded at me. Then he turned and walked out.

"I feel totally ridiculous," I said to Harriet.

"Kase." She pointed to her floral nightgown tucked into her jeans. We both laughed. While she went to get the car, I got dressed. I walked out into the hallway with discharge papers in hand. The doctor came down the hall. "Take care," he said as we passed each other.

"Thanks." I kept walking toward the waiting room.

"Hey," he called.

I stopped and turned around.

"Have you been under any stress lately?"

I leaned into the wall. He stood there, waiting for an answer. "Oh . . . I don't know . . ." I thought about his patients in the other rooms. "Maybe a little." I rubbed my eyes. "You know, the usual."

He studied me for a moment more, and I offered him a slight smile.

On the drive back to the Harbor we called my parents. "I'll get you in with my doctor first thing in the morning," my dad said. "Get down here early." The clock on the car radio glowed 3:24 in an eerie blue light. I thought about the couple hours of sleep I'd get before the kids woke as usual at 6:00 A.M.

The next day, I met my parents in the parking lot of their

doctor's office. Mom came over to the car, and I rolled down the window. "How could that emergency doctor say there's nothing wrong with you?" she said. "You look terrible."

"Thanks, Mom," I looked down at her tattered sweat-pants and flip-flops. "So do you."

"I know," she looked around. "Let me in the car before someone I know sees me." I got out of the driver's seat, and she took my place. "Dad's gonna stay with you," she said. "I'll take the kids back to the house." I opened the back door and kissed both kids goodbye. Dad was standing behind me. He hadn't shaved and his shirt was a little untucked on one side. I watched the car drive off. "Let's get in there, Arnold," he said, putting an arm around my shoulder. "The doc's doin' me a real favor squeezing you in this morning." Dad and I started walking toward the office building. "I got a hold of Lee at work," he said.

"What did you tell him?"

"I told him you had some chest pain in the night." I nodded. "What'd he say?"

"He was upset and asked if he should come up. I told him we'd call him when we got through here and knew more."

Dad's doctor ran a bunch of tests with fancy names that I was too tired to remember. After my chest x-rays, we were sitting in the waiting room, when the door opened behind me.

My dad rose. "Lee," he said. "How the hell'd you get here?"

I didn't care how he got there. In a matter of seconds I was across the room and wrapped in his arms. Burying my face deep in his chest, I breathed in the smell of his blue button-down shirt. He leaned down and kissed the top of my head. "You okay, babe?"

"I don't know," I shook my head. "I don't know anymore."

Dad walked over. "Lee, you're a magician." He patted him on the back. "One minute I'm on the phone with you, the next you're walking through the door. How'd you do it?"

"I couldn't just sit there, so I left the office, took a cab to Logan, and hopped on the next flight up."

My dad raised his eyebrows. "How much did that ticket run ya?"

Lee and I laughed. "It wasn't cheap . . ." He looked down at me. "But what else could I do?" He squeezed my shoulder.

My dad shook his head in amazement. He was always on an endless pursuit to find discount airfares.

Dad's doctor called us back into his office to report that all the tests looked normal. "You most likely had an anxiety attack," he said.

Anxiety attack? An anxiety attack meant sweaty palms and a rapid heart rate, not the feelings of a heart attack or stroke. But the doctor said it was quite common for an anxiety attack to feel just like that.

On the car ride to my parents I slumped in the backseat. Inside I screamed at myself, *You're ridiculous. You're weak and frail and feeble. You're pathetic.*

At my parents I slept for a couple hours. When I woke up, we got back in the car and drove up to the Harbor. We wanted to go home, but I'd left all our stuff up there. Lee had been in the clothes he'd worn to work, so he'd borrowed a t-shirt and shorts from my dad.

That night, after we'd put the kids to bed, Lee and I sat

on the cottage steps looking out at the water. "I can't do this, babe," I said. "I can't take care of these kids."

"Yes you can," Lee said. "You're strong."

"*Strong*. I don't even know what that means anymore."

Ever since Andie was born everyone had been telling me how strong I was. Whenever I questioned my ability to raise Andie, I would repeat back to myself what I'd heard. "You're so strong." But, I didn't really understand what it meant to be strong. Or perhaps, I misunderstood. I thought being strong meant being stoic, standing proud to receive whatever news came my way, with my back straight and my shoulders squared, unwavering in my beliefs, like the great skyscrapers that stand confidently over city skylines.

But I learned that architects intentionally design flexibility into those tall buildings. Without the ability to move with changing wind patterns and volatile ground shifts, the buildings would come crashing down—like me. I had only been able to stand for so long. Without flexibility and an ability to sway, I'd come crumbling down. I was at my weakest and most powerless, and I was pretty sure I couldn't be rebuilt. And like a fallen building that crowds gather around, I was wreckage for all to see.

Yet it wound up being there, in that heap, that I would discover the true meaning of strength; not in picking myself up, but in staying down and letting go. Surrendering to the fact that I couldn't go on, I would eventually realize that strength and vulnerability share the same gene. They coil around one another like basic strands of human DNA. To be vulnerable became my biggest strength.

Back at home, where I could breathe again, our days were slow. I allowed myself to be tired, napping when the kids napped and climbing into bed at night right after they did.

From my bed one morning, I called Aunt Mimi, mom's twin, who was a therapist in Colorado. She put on her professional therapist's hat and explained the body's physical reaction to a buildup of stress and trauma. She pointed out that much of my anxiety probably wasn't just from what we'd been through, but from what we were anticipating going through: *the still pending ostomy reversal surgery*.

I'd already read that the greatest fear of a preemie parent was to have their child back in the hospital. Mimi and I talked about how it felt to know the event was coming, but not know when. The *not knowing* was killing me. We wanted to move forward with our lives, but the surgeon held all the cards. Waiting for this surgery was like having a tack in my shoe; I was always aware of it, and when I stepped forward it lodged deeper in.

"Why are you giving that doctor all the control?" Mimi asked.

"I don't know," I said. "I didn't really know I was."

Mimi suggested I call another surgeon.

"But this guy saved Andie's life," I said.

"And he's ruining yours."

"I'm afraid that if we choose another surgeon, the original doctor will be angry and somehow screw up the surgery." I waited for Mimi to laugh, but she didn't.

"That sounds like a pretty normal fear to me," she said.

I couldn't believe how much better I felt.

Finally, I picked up a pen and notebook from my bedside table, and Mimi and I came up with a plan to rebuild.

1. *Call Andie's nurses, Marcia and Yvonne, and ask them to recommend another surgeon.*
2. *Contact the new surgeon, explain the situation, and set up a consultation.*

"OPERATION TAKE BACK CONTROL," I wrote across the top of the page.

And I did. Later that day I found myself calling the alternative surgeon's office and setting a date to meet him in person. As I was chopping carrots for dinner, the phone rang. It was the receptionist calling from the office of Andie's original surgeon. They were ready to schedule Andie's surgery. *Well, imagine that.* I pictured the alternative surgeon's receptionist walking down the hall and poking her head around this surgeon's door. "You know we just received a phone call . . ."

I stood in the kitchen holding the knife in my hand. Part of me wanted to tell the receptionist, to tell the doctor, to go fuck himself. But the other part of me wanted Andie in and out of that hospital with the surgery over.

So I said yes, we would accept the surgery date of October 9, 2001, just a little over a month away.

23

Gardens

✦

A s I was emerging from my figurative pile of rubble, our friend Mike was buried beneath a real one in lower Manhattan on September eleventh, 2001. His memorial service took place in a small chapel in Connecticut two days before Andie's surgery. His daughter, Sydney, who shares Tucker's birthday, walked down the aisle wearing a white cotton sweater with an American flag knit across the front. He was Canadian.

Following the memorial, we picked the kids up at Sandy's house, the same Sandy who took care of Tuck during our ski getaway. She met us at the door with Andie in her arms, wrapped in a dark green bath towel. "Her ostomy bag fell off," she said, looking embarrassed. Lee took Andie from her arms. "I am so sorry," I kept telling her, as Lee carried Andie and the ostomy supplies into the other room.

On the drive home Lee said, "Two more days and no more ostomy bag." My stomach clenched, and the list of surgery risks began swirling through my head: internal bleeding, infection, reaction to anesthesia . . . My mind began to move into panic mode. I reached down for the bag at my feet and drew out the book my friend Nancy had recommended—*Prepare for Surgery, Heal Faster* by Peggy Huddleston. I turned to the page I'd marked in chapter two. Glancing back at the sleeping kids, I quietly read out loud, "When worries about the operation pop into your mind, switch them to pictures of the healed result, as if you were changing the channel on a TV." Lee squeezed my hand. "Thank God for that book," he said. The next morning I met Karen for my final appointment before Andie's surgery. "I want to do some muscle testing on you," she told me, "to see if you're ready for Andie's surgery."

"I feel ready," I told her.

She nodded. "Yeah, but we want to make sure you're *really* ready on all levels: physical, emotional, mental, and spiritual."

I lay flat on my back on Karen's table and held my arm straight out to the side. Gently, she placed her hand on my outstretched arm. I knew the drill. She'd ask me specific questions, and I'd watch my arm either hold firm, meaning yes, or fall limply to my side, for no.

Karen gave my arm a tender squeeze and began, "Is Kasey fully prepared for Andie's surgery tomorrow?" she asked.

As my mind said yes, I watched my arm fall to my side.

"Does she have lingering fears about the surgery?" Karen asked.

My arm and my mind both said yes.

"Is this still Kasey's fear of Andie dying?"

I didn't dare to guess which way that one would go.

"No," Karen said, as my arm fell.

Her gaze moved past my head to the corner of the room, and her face went still as she thought of her next question. Then her eyebrows shot up, and she turned back to me. "Is this Kasey's fear of her *own* death?" she asked.

What's that got to do with anything, I thought, but watched as my arm held steady. *Yes.*

Karen let my arm rest on the table. She pushed her hair back over her shoulder and gently placed her hand on my wrist. "How are you going to die?" she asked.

"*What?*" I let out a shocked laugh.

"How are you going to die?" she asked again.

I propped up on my elbows. "How am *I* supposed to know?"

"You do know," Karen said. I looked at her. Her silver earrings glanced in the light. "Will you be driving a car at 100 miles an hour and slam into a tree?"

I pictured a flashy red sports car racing down a windy narrow road and cringed. "No way," I said.

"Then how?" she asked.

"God, Karen, I don't know." I stared out the window at the birch trees swaying in the wind. Then I surprised myself by saying, "Cancer."

"Where?" she asked without hesitation.

I watched my hands clasp my chest.

"Ah, so you're going to die of cancer to pay back for all of the suffering Andie has gone through?"

My mind couldn't make sense of what she was saying, but some deeper part of me knew exactly what she meant. "Yes."

"No," she said.

"No?"

"That's not how you're going to die. Not unless you want it to be." She gave my arm a squeeze.

"Well, I don't."

"Then tell me how." She drew out each word slowly, "Tell me how you want to die?"

I closed my eyes. When I was eight I'd cried myself to sleep for months imagining my parents suddenly dying. Death was black, dark, and deep. Death was terrifying. But in Karen's office, lying on that narrow massage table warmed by the heating pad beneath, my gloomy canvas of death was suddenly exposed to light. Shadowy colors changed before my eyes. Black became violet. Death became fields of lavender and wandering pea-stone garden paths. It became an unveiling, revealing joy, luminous and serene. Death became a beginning.

"I will be old and tired and beautiful," I said aloud. I kept my eyes closed and saw myself in a garden, wearing a broad straw hat, holding a basket full of scented lavender, my tall frame slightly stooped and my skin more freckled with age. "I will be full and complete." I blew out a long, full breath.

When I opened my eyes, Karen was looking down at me with a big smile on her face.

"Well, my dear," she slid her hand under my shoulder and helped me to a sitting position, "It looks like both you and your daughter are ready for the surgery."

◆

We arrived at Children's Hospital early the next day. They had to prep Andie's intestines for surgery first. We'd already done some prep. For several weeks, we'd been squeezing stool from Andie's ostomy bag into a diaper and then putting the diaper back on her. "The diaper rash will be severe," the nurse had warned during our pre-surgery appointment. "It can last a good six to eight weeks. Remember, her bum has never seen stool before. You want to toughen it up to avoid open sores that could lead to an infection."

I thought putting a dirty diaper *back on a child* was the most unnatural thing a parent could do. But the day before the surgery, I had to do something even more unnatural. I had to purposely deny my eleven-month-old daughter food. Her intestinal tract had to be completely empty before the surgery could be performed.

Andie wore a hospital gown with teddy bears all over it and sat in the hospital bed in a double room on the third floor. Three different children would occupy the other bed during her weeklong stay. An IV stretched from her arm to the bag of nutrients hanging over her head. Every few minutes she willed her big hazel eyes away from the *Barney* video and pointed to her mouth.

Andie loved to eat. At dinnertime we called her our little Hoover. She devoured every new food that came her way. *How will we ever get through this?* I thought, and shamefully looked away when she begged for food.

I thought things couldn't get any worse until two nurses appeared in the doorway announcing it was time for Andie's first enema. "Gotta make sure she's all cleaned out," the one on the right said with a smile. A memory of the week I'd spent at summer camp with the stomach bug when I was 10 flashed to mind. While the other kids roasted marshmallows and sang campfire songs, I spent the week in the infirmary with the wretched old nurse who crushed penicillin pills for

me to swallow and refused to call my parents. When I finally
stopped throwing up after five days she said, "Now we gotta
make sure you're all cleaned out." I learned what an enema
was and spent the last two days at camp sitting on the toilet
shitting out brown water.

As the Children's nurses crossed the threshold, I instinc-
tively stepped closer to Andie's bed. "We just need to take
her to a room down the hall."

I looked at Lee with wide eyes. "We'll go with you," he
said.

＋

The room was small with tiled walls and a metal table in
the center. Lee gently laid Andie on her back on the table.
Her little toes curled away from the cold table. One of the
nurses tugged her gown up and started removing her ostomy
bag. "What are you doing?" I asked, horrified she was taking
off the bag we'd put on only yesterday. She looked up, but
her fingers continued to pull back the adhesive and plastic
from Andie's stomach. "We have to go in through the ostomy
opening," she said casually. I gripped the side of the metal
table. The other nurse walked over with a long black tube
that looked like a poisonous snake. I couldn't believe what I
was seeing. Every fiber of my maternal being thought it was
totally wrong. "That's a girl," the nurse with the tube said to
Andie, as the other pulled apart the slimy opening of Andie's
stoma. I watched the black tube go in. The nurse holding
the tube took a step back to stretch out the several feet of
tubing, while the other slowly fed it in. "She's so good," she

said looking up at me. Then Andie whimpered and reached toward her belly. "Can you hold her arms, Dad?" the nurse asked. Lee did.

An enormous scream was pulsing at the back of my throat, and I let out a low moan. It sounded more like a growl. "Maybe it would be easier for you to wait in the hallway, Mom," the nurse said.

I looked at Lee. "Go, babe," he said. "I'm with her." I took one last look at the feet of tubing still to go and nearly ran from the room.

In the hallway, I stood against the wall, slowly banging my head, hating myself for not being stronger. About 30 minutes later, they emerged from the room. Lee carried Andie in his arms, her light eyebrows arched high above her startled eyes. She clung to Lee's neck. One of the nurses put her hand on my shoulder. "She is such a good baby. She never even cried." I tried to smile, as I wiped the tears off my cheeks.

The nurses returned four or five more times that day. Lee dutifully picked up Andie each time and followed them out the door while I stayed behind in the room, staring at my shoes.

The next morning finally arrived. I couldn't sit still, so I flitted around the room taking pictures. I took several of Andie and a few of her ostomy bag. "Goodbye, ostomy," I said in a high, squeaky voice. In the pre-op room, Andie sat in the last bed in a long row of maybe six or seven others. Her surgeon stood at the end of her bed, his reading glasses perched on the end of his nose, reviewing Andie's paperwork. I snapped a picture of him. He startled when the flash went off and looked up from his clipboard. "Sorry," I smiled. He smiled back. His necktie had pictures of tiny children lined up in rows. "I like your tie," I said, but I really wanted to say, *Please don't let my daughter die.*

We stood next to Andie's bed waiting for the anesthesiologist to arrive. I clasped the index cards on which I'd written healing statements, another trick from *Prepare for Surgery, Heal Faster.* I read what we'd written on the card and noticed that my sweaty fingers blurred a couple of the words. *During this operation you will feel comfortable and safe. Your body is strong. You are so loved.* The second card, for when the surgery was over, read, *Your operation has been a success. Following this surgery your intestinal tract will be clear and flow with ease. You will heal well and completely.* Lee watched me reading the cards. "Do you think the anesthesiologist is going to think we're total whack jobs?" I asked.

"Probably," Lee said. Then he picked up Andie's little pink hand in his. "But do we really care?"

I looked at the IV taped to Andie's tiny wrist and shook my head.

The double doors swung open and a tall guy with curly brown shoulder-length hair walked in. He and Andie's surgeon shook hands. The surgeon turned to us and introduced him as the anesthesiologist. He had gorgeous blue eyes and a strong handshake. I imagined he was a rock climber and ate all organic food from a co-op grocery. I held out the index cards and asked if he'd read each card five times as Andie was going under and coming out of the surgery. "Cool," he said, pushing a brown curl out of his eye. "Research is showing this stuff really works. Speeds up healing. Good for you guys." And then he walked across the room to meet his other patients.

Not long afterward, a surgical nurse arrived and said it was time to take Andie. "This is it," Lee said.

I kissed Andie on her cheeks and lips and forehead and breathed in the smell of her soft, downy hair. I whispered in her ear, "I love you, Andie Lou." She grabbed a fist full of my hair and pulled me closer.

Lee leaned in, and rested his forehead on Andie's other cheek. "You are so strong, Andie. We'll be waiting for you. I love you so much." We stayed that way until the nurse cleared her throat. When we stood up, Andie's big eyes looked stunned, and she reached out toward me. I held her hand in mine. The nurse released the brake on the hospital bed. As she started rolling the bed away from me, Andie's fingers slid out of mine. She opened her mouth as if to say, "Mama." My breath caught in my throat. I started to follow, but Lee grabbed my arm and held me back. We watched the nurse's back as she rolled Andie away from us. I strained to hear any sounds coming from her, but heard none. Still, my heart could hear her silent screams.

I sat in the waiting room on a hard plastic chair beside Lee. I had my water and my Rescue Remedy, along with my earphones and my guided imagery tape. Leaning my head back, I visualized Andie dancing above her body as the team of surgeons hovered over her. She held hands and danced with a circle of angels, our friend Mike, my grandmother, and Daniel. There was so much music and laughter and joy in my vision, I wanted to get up and dance with them.

I was so lost in my own world that I had no idea how

much time went by before Lee nudged me. I opened my eyes. The surgeon stood before us. His green scrubs snapped my mind back to reality. "The surgery was a success." Lee and I stood up, and in the midst of our teary thank yous, the doctor said, "Oh, I took her appendix out while I was in there." As we followed him down the hall to the recovery room I whispered to Lee. "Did we want her appendix out?"

"Too late now," he whispered back.

We stayed in the hospital five more days, because we weren't allowed to go home until Andie pooped. They had to be sure her excrement could navigate its way through her entire intestinal tract. Until she pooped, she couldn't eat. The *Barney* marathon was no longer distracting her from hunger. I feared she'd chew her big blue pacifier in half.

Waiting for Andie to poop was torture. In her desperation to eat, nothing kept her entertained or happy. We read her books, played with puppets, and walked her around the hospital in her stroller with the IV cart trailing behind. Still, she fussed and cried and tugged at the Velcro sleeves covering the IV tube on her wrist.

Marcia came over from the NICU and gave Andie a "Get Well" balloon from the gift shop. Karen McCarthy came in and did a healing. She asked the nurse if there was anyone on staff available to do Reiki. The nurse said she thought so and promised to look into it, but no one ever came. My mom brought Tucker to visit. He climbed into bed next to Andie, hugging her tightly. "Hi Andie," he said. "Whatcha doin'?"

Lee and I took turns leaving the hospital for walks. He discovered a bar at the hotel next door. I discovered the Isabella Stewart Gardner Museum.

I arrived late on Sunday afternoon, a half hour before closing. The plaque at the entrance told me Isabella Stewart Gardner, a Boston socialite, had opened her home as a museum in 1903. She'd spent over 30 years traveling the world, amassing a huge collection of fine art. "It's too late for the galleries," the young man behind the desk said, "but you can visit the courtyard if you like."

When I walked in and saw the beauty of the three-story Italianate courtyard, I stopped breathing. I couldn't believe I'd found a magical garden paradise in the middle of Boston, just around the corner from Children's Hospital. Sitting down on the steps, I looked up at the stone arches, the perfectly trimmed palm trees, the potted jade plants, and the green grass surrounding the mosaic tile floor. In silence and gratitude, I sat there until a security guard tapped me on the shoulder and told me it was time to leave. While I was following him out, I turned one last time to take in the incredible foliage, and vowed someday I'd share it with my daughter.

On our fourth poopless evening, Lee tried to convince me to visit his bar. The offer was tempting, but Andie hadn't been left alone once since we'd arrived at the hospital, and I was nervous about going. Lee took the magazine out of my hand and pointed to Andie. She was sound asleep with her head tipped back and her mouth open. He flashed me the smile I'd never been able to resist. "Since the day I met you," I said as we walked down the hall to the nurse's station, "you could talk me into anything." Lee squeezed my hand and told the nurse we were going out for "a walk."

A bottle of Bud never tasted so good. "I *love* this beer," I said to Lee. "I love *you*." I kissed him square on the mouth.

When we returned to the hospital, we found an inconsolable Andie crying in a nurse's arms. I glared at Lee and took Andie from the nurse, hoping she couldn't smell the beer on my breath.

The next morning—day five—we were all sitting around watching Barney lead a parade across the screen when, drum roll please . . . Andie pooped. *Hallelujah.* We could finally feed our daughter, go home, and get on with the rest of our lives.

✦

I sat on the bed, watching Lee change Andie's diaper. Just as the nurse demonstrated in the hospital, he slathered a thick layer of diaper cream on her bum. "Like cream cheese on a bagel," I said. He rolled his eyes as he sprinkled on the special powder meant to absorb any rash-aggravating moisture.

"When do you think the rash will start?" I asked.

"Is that the fiftieth or sixtieth time you've asked me in the past week?" he said as he picked her up.

A week later, he was changing Andie's diaper again, when I started to ask, "Do you think it's possible that . . ." but he cut me off.

"Don't say it," he warned.

"Oh that's right," I rolled my eyes. "Sorry, Mr. Superstitious."

"I'm not superstitious," he said, kissing Andie on both her cheeks.

"Oh no," I said. "You're not superstitious." And reminded him about watching the Red Sox during a recent winning streak on our tiny 13-inch kitchen TV because he feared his move to the living room would somehow bring about their downfall.

"They won didn't they?" He picked Andie up and jiggled her on his hip.

I nodded. "Yeah," I said. "They did."

My mind wandered back to the hospital and the healing Karen performed. I thought of *Prepare for Surgery, Heal Faster* and the visualizations we'd been practicing. Not only did Andie not have a rash two weeks post-surgery, there wasn't a single red bump anywhere on her little bum.

After another week, we were back at Children's Hospital for her follow-up. It was hard to hide our smiles as the nurse pulled back Andie's diaper and covered her mouth with her hand. She looked from me to Lee and back again. "There's no rash," she said.

I nodded. Lee rocked back and forth on his toes with his arms crossed over his chest.

The nurse bent down again, squinting to get a closer look. "I've been a skin therapist for 19 years and have never seen anything like this. What did you do?"

Gathering an excited breath, I prepared to tell her all about energy healing, imagining the impact our story would have on surgical patients worldwide, but Lee pinched the back of my arm, warning me to stay quiet.

I'd jumped into the world of alternative medicine with both feet and seen firsthand how amazing it was. Lee supported the work, but he believed his job was to constantly question and play devil's advocate. As I dove in, he sat high in the lifeguard chair, making sure I wasn't swimming too far from shore and taking our kids with me. Eventually, he'd wade in and swim right along beside us, but that would be sometime later.

When the nurse looked up at us again, I gave Lee's hand a squeeze and said, "Just lucky, I guess."

24

Shoes

◆

ANDIE WAS A PINK FLOPPY-EARED BUNNY for her first Halloween. Tucker made his own "Super Tucker" costume out of dark blue long johns, a white turtleneck with a big "T" on the front, and a red cape. After Lee strapped the kids into the double jogger stroller to take them trick or treating, I passed him a diaper to put in the basket beneath. "It is so nice not to have to haul around that bag of ostomy supplies," he said.

When Andie's early intervention coordinator, Margaret, came for her scheduled visit she marveled at Andie's smooth belly. "You must be so glad to have the surgery behind you!" she said, pulling toys out of her big green duffle bag.

"Yeah," I answered, but I didn't feel as much relief as I had expected. Instead, I felt like I was still waiting for something. I watched Margaret playfully pinch the toe on one of Andie's little denim sneakers. Andie giggled. I studied Andie's shoes. *That's it*, I thought, *I'm waiting for the other shoe to drop.*

Apparently the origination of that shoe-dropping expression had nothing to do with an exhausted, confused mother of a preemie. As the story goes, a road-weary traveler arrived late one night to a boarding house. Sitting on the edge of his bed, he unlaced one of his shoes and let it fall loudly to the floor. Suddenly aware of the other sleeping residents, he quietly removed the other shoe and placed it down gently on the floor. Then he climbed into bed and soon fell asleep. Sometime later he was startled awake by a voice calling from the room below. "Well, drop the other one already. I can't sleep waiting for *the other shoe to drop.*"

"I'm plagued by shoes," I told Karen McCarthy at my next appointment. She laughed and handed me a glass of water. "What's that supposed to mean?"

I sipped the water and set the plastic cup down on the table. "Well, I figured out why I still feel so jittery and unsettled even though Andie's surgery is over," I said, leaning back in the chair. "I'm still waiting for something to happen."

"The other shoe to drop?" Karen guessed.

"Exactly." I fingered the toe of my fleece sock. "I also hate having to ask people to leave their shoes at the door."

Ever since Andie arrived home from the hospital, asking people to remove their shoes had caused me great distress. My mother, physically hours away, stood directly behind me, shaking her head, outraged by the greeting I'd offered my visitors. I found myself saying, "I'm so sorry, I know this seems rude, but would you please mind taking off your shoes? The doctors and nurses have stressed how vulnerable Andie is to illness and shoes carry quite a lot of germs and toxins, and with her spending time crawling on the floor . . ." and on and on I would go.

When I tried to explain my pussyfooting around to Karen, she came at me like a mean old stiletto. "Are you kidding me?" she said. "You're worried about asking people to take off their shoes?"

I hunched my shoulders and looked down at the carpeted floor, and Karen cooled off a bit. Pointing at Andie, asleep in her car seat beside me, she said, "Kasey, we're talking about your daughter's life here." I looked at Andie's long lashes resting on her cheeks. "Your daughter doesn't have her own voice," Karen said. "You must speak for her. She is relying on you to say what she cannot." She sat on the edge of her chair and spoke slowly and clearly, "You must find, and use, your voice." She placed a hand on my knee. "This is just one of the many life lessons Andie has come to teach you."

I lifted my shoulders and let them fall. "Well when you put it that way," I said and we both laughed. Andie startled in her sleep, but didn't wake.

Before we left, I practiced using my new voice. Standing in front of the skeleton in Karen's office I said, "Please leave your shoes outside the door," in a strong, unwavering voice.

"Yes," Karen said. "That's it." She'd made it so simple. Why had I made it so difficult?

At home, when I heard a knock on the door, Karen's voice echoed in my ears. *This is your daughter's life . . . she doesn't have a voice.* I still felt uncomfortable, but I did it.

I noticed I was starting to use my newfound voice other times, too. The doctor's office presented many opportunities. I expressed concerns about germs in the waiting room and asked to be taken directly to the exam room. When the receptionist rolled her eyes, I told her we'd be happy to wait outside in the parking lot.

When Andie's primary doctor, the infamous "preemie spotter," told me there was a nationwide shortage of the flu vaccine and there was none available for Andie because he had *forgotten she was a preemie*, I really found my voice. I told the doctor that I would persist until a flu vaccine was found, and he pushed up the sleeves of his fine knit sweater and said that the only possible way was if he took the vaccine away from another baby. Or in his exact words, "I will have to rob Peter to pay Paul."

I clutched the exam table and stared directly into his eyes. "Are you suggesting I feel guilty about putting the needs of my own child first?" I asked, knowing it was time to find Andie a new doctor.

My newfound voice taught me to question, rather than simply accept. My new voice offered me power, control, and a chance to stop playing the victim.

It seemed that once this learning opportunity emerged, the lessons for it repeated over and over again. Like an old school marm, the Universe kept offering little pop quizzes, ensuring that I'd fully integrated the lesson.

And just when I thought I'd finally mastered the tutorial of finding and using my voice, what came next would be the equivalent of my hardest final exam.

25

Second Chances

✦

BY LATE NOVEMBER, Andie had turned two and chipped away the last pieces of mortar surrounding my heart. My walls had come down, and she'd climbed inside.

Her second birthday brought tremendous relief. My parents and John and Lollie came for Thanksgiving and stayed through the weekend to celebrate. We tied big yellow balloons to Andie's chair and strung streamers across the kitchen. Everyone wore coned party hats. Lee and Tuck stood by her side, while I snapped pictures of Andie pursing her lips before she blew out her candles. When Tucker leaned in and tried to help her, she pushed him back. "No, Tucker," she said. "Mine." Everyone roared with laughter. She'd made it so far and done so well. It was time to live again.

When December arrived, I hung wreathes, put candles in every window, and played Christmas music while I did the dishes at night. "Kasey's got her groove back," Lee teased, swatting me with a dishtowel.

"Hey," he caught me by the hand one night when I'd just turned down the volume on a Vivaldi Christmas concert. The kids were sleeping. He drew me onto his lap on the living room couch. "Come with me to Colorado." He kissed me on the neck. I laughed. "And what will we do with the kids?" He bit my ear softly. "We have a thousand people ready to babysit." He ran his finger up my spine. "You can sleep all morning while I'm in meetings, and we'll ski all afternoon." I shook my head. "I don't know, babe. I'm scared to leave her." He touched my face. "I know," he whispered. "But she's okay, and we need to remember each other." I closed my eyes and kissed him back, feeling the rough stubble of his cheek. We'd been so busy caring for our children that we lost sight of our needs as a couple. I'd always believed mothers should put their own needs first, and then when Andie was born, all my rules changed. But she wasn't a helpless baby anymore. She was a sparkly two-year-old who loved to turn on the stereo and run around the house, wearing nothing but Lee's baseball cap on backwards. Lee was right, it was time to move forward. "Okay," I whispered in his ear. "I'll go."

◆

In early January Andie began rubbing her right ear. She had a runny nose. Our trip was only a few weeks away so I took her to the doctor's office just to be safe. The young doctor on call was dressed the way I had in seventh grade: a white turtleneck with little snowflake patterns, wide wale corduroys, and her hair clipped to the side in a barrette. Tiny chips of the silver laminate had peeled off her barrette and speckled her hair. She raised her eyebrows when she lifted Andie's thick manila file off the counter. As I did with every other new medical provider, I took her through Andie's long and unusual birth history.

When she placed her stethoscope on Andie's bare chest, Andie reached out to touch one of the snowflakes. "You like snow?" she asked and turned her head to listen. I watched her eyes narrow. It was very quiet in the office. The wall clock ticked. Andie scratched a spot on her shoulder. "Hmm," the doctor said, moving the stethoscope a little to the right. Her hands were cracked and dry. I could tell she chewed her nails. "I hear a little something in her lungs." She brought the stethoscope to the other side of Andie's back. "I'm going to order some x-rays," she said. My palms started to sweat. I wanted to call Lee, but I told myself I could do this. I'll call him when the x-rays come back, I told myself.

The x-rays were clear. I went home, assured that Andie's lungs were in fine shape. *Colorado, here we come.*

The next morning I was cleaning up after breakfast when the phone rang.

I immediately recognized the doctor's voice from the day before. "The radiologist who reviewed the x-rays actually saw a little spot on Andie's lungs."

I wiped my hands on the dishtowel hanging from the stove. "Okay," I said.

"Just to be on the safe side," the doctor said, "why don't you come in at the end of the week for a re-check."

On Friday I got Tucker off to preschool, grabbed a snack bag of Cheerios, and headed to the doctor's office with Andie. There'd been other days when we'd had to wait at the office, but that morning was ridiculous. We waited and waited. Andie kept resting her head on my lap. I looked up at the clock. Thirty minutes had passed. Taking Andie's hand, I walked up to the desk. The receptionist looked at me over the frames of her reading glasses. "You'll be called soon," she said.

After 45 minutes I wanted to take Andie home. "The doctor is dealing with an emergency situation," the receptionist said when I asked. "We'll call you in as soon as we can." She slid the glass window closed.

After almost an hour, a nurse finally called Andie's name. By then Andie was too exhausted to walk, so I picked her up in my arms. Her soft blond head nestled into my shoulder, as I followed the nurse down the hall toward the exam room. Just as we got to the door, we heard a commotion from the end the hall. A group of EMTs burst out, wheeling a little girl on a stretcher. Outside I saw an ambulance, it's red lights flashing.

"The emergency?" I asked.

The nurse nodded.

Moments after sitting down in the exam room, the nurse put Andie's pointer finger in an oxygen meter, and her eyes widened as she read the numbers. She bit her lower lip, glanced at me, then quickly left the room. When she returned, she was carrying a machine and an oxygen mask. She put the oxygen mask over Andie's face. Two other nurses and a doctor came into the room.

"What's going on?" I could feel that bitter panic rising in my throat.

"She's having some trouble breathing," the doctor said and then she left the room again.

I thought about how long we'd been sitting in the waiting room. "Is this another emergency?" I asked.

The nurses looked up from checking Andie's blood pressure and heartbeat. "Yes," they answered in unison.

The doctor came back in. "An ambulance is on its way," she said.

"*Ambulance?*" I looked from her to Andie to the nurses, my heartbeat sped up. "Medical stuff," I said, "is really my husband's thing." I backed up. "I don't really—" My shoulder bumped into the phone on the wall. "Can I use this?" I asked the doctor.

I dialed Lee's work number. My fingers were shaking.

"You have to dial 9 to get an outside line," said the nurse holding Andie.

I held the phone to my ear and listened to the ringing noise. "Please be there," I kept whispering.

"Hello," Lee answered.

"Oh my God, Lee, Andie's having trouble breathing . . . an ambulance is coming . . . we have to go to the ER . . . Lee, I can't do this . . . I can't do this."

I looked over at Andie, cradled in a nurse's lap with a clear plastic mask covering her face. *Please God, please don't take her from me.* She was wearing her yellow sweater with the white faux fur collar. It was my favorite. The phone was shaking in my hand. *Please God.*

"Kasey, listen to me," Lee said. "You've gotta step up to the plate. I'll be there as soon as I can, but you can do this." I didn't answer. "Do you hear me?"

"Yes," I whispered into the phone. The EMTs were coming down the hallway. "I have to go."

I put the phone back on the wall. The first EMT walked in. I recognized him from the local coffee shop. The nurses and EMTs strapped Andie onto a gurney, the mask still covering her mouth and nose. Andie's eyes went wide when they started wheeling the gurney backwards out of the room. I stepped around the doctor and moved next to the gurney. As we moved down the hall, my shoe caught the heel of the EMT in front of me three times.

Andie's body looked tiny on the ambulance gurney. Later I would wish I had sat next to her, touched her, told her that she was going to be alright. But I didn't. Instead, I leaned as far away from her as possible. We passed our local grocery store as the sirens blared. "Anyone need a quart of milk?" I asked, trying to distract my fears. The guys glanced at me. They laughed politely.

We arrived at the emergency entrance of the closest hospital. Andie was wheeled into a room. The same young girl who'd just left the office in an ambulance was lying on the bed near the window. The girl was older than I'd thought. "Six," the mom said. "Two," I told her when she asked. *Two was supposed to be safe*, I thought.

That mom was calm. I told her how scared I was. "She'll be okay," she said.

Lee arrived. X-rays were taken and a young doctor on rounds from Children's Hospital was assigned to Andie's case. He leaned against the door frame of Andie's room and hooked his thumb in the front pocket of his jeans. We stood by Andie's bed, watching him. "So the nasal swab tells us she's got RSV," he said.

Lee shook his head. "*Fucking RSV*," he said. The doctors had warned us about Respiratory Syncytial Virus, which is very common and very contagious. In most healthy children, it acts like a cold, but in infants and preemies, RSV can cause major breathing problems. Synagis, a shot that can be used every month during the fall and winter to minimize the chance of getting RSV, is quite costly and insurance companies often fight coverage. We were both thinking about the battle we'd had with our insurance company the year before when they tried to deny Andie Synagis. We didn't even try to get it that second year.

"Her x-rays have me pretty freaked," the doctor said.

My knees started to go. I held fast to the bed rail.

The doctor ran his fingers through his hair. "There isn't really anything we can do." He sighed. "It's gonna be up to her."

We looked down at Andie. Her big green eyes stared back at us over the oxygen mask. Lee cradled the top of her head with his hand. "It's just gonna depend on how much she wants to fight this." The doctor stood up straighter. "And she'll have to be moved to a hospital with an ICU unit," he said.

The other shoe had dropped and I ran out of the room, down the long hospital corridor, and through the exit door before it even hit the floor. Standing outside, I gasped for breath. Two nurses and a guy who must have been an orderly stood there smoking. The orderly nodded to me. I leaned against the cold brick wall and pulled my cell phone out of my pocket. Then I called every person in our family. "I don't know what to do," I told them over and over. "She might not make it." All they could do was panic from farther away.

After I'd called everyone in our family, I called my yoga

teacher, Nancy. When she said hello, I pictured her sitting on the Indian rug next to the jade tree in her front living room. "Andie has RSV," I said. "They don't know if she'll make it." She didn't ask for details. "Kasey, listen to me carefully." Her voice was calm. "I want you to put the phone down and go back in there. Put your hands on Andie's chest and *breathe* for her. Go. Now," she said.

I closed my phone. The smokers were gone. I stood impatiently in front of the sliding glass doors, waiting for them to open. Then I ran all the way back down that long corridor and through the door of her room. Lee looked up with wide eyes. I pulled a chair to the side of the bed and placed my hands on Andie's small chest. She reached out to me and I lifted her onto my lap. Lee adjusted the mask and covered her with a blanket. Her body felt so light, like a bag full of feathers. "Oh, Andie," I said. "I'm here now. I won't leave you." I spread my fingers across her thin, bony back and took a long, slow breath, nuzzling my head against her ear. "You're so strong, baby," I said. "You can fight this." I leaned back in the chair and closed my eyes. Andie's whole body rose and fell on my chest with every breath she and I took together.

The ER doctor walked in the room. "Okay," he said. "The plan has changed." He mumbled something about bed shortages at the big hospitals. "We'll admit her here instead." Our nurse-practitioner friend, Stephanie, who had arrived a few minutes before, was sitting in the corner out of his line of sight, and I saw her shake her head from side to side.

I remembered what Karen had said in her office that day when I told her I hated asking people to take their shoes off. I cleared my throat.

"Can I speak to you out in the hall?" I asked.

The doctor's eyebrows shot up. "Sure," he said. Passing Andie to Lee, I whispered to her, "I'll be right back." Then I pulled myself up taller, imagined I had on my kick-some-ass cowboy boots, and followed the doctor out into the hall.

"We were told our child needs to be in a hospital with an ICU." Even to myself I sounded like a lawyer in a courtroom. "We will *not* have her admitted to this hospital. You will have to find her a bed at one of the bigger hospitals." I took a breath. "Nothing else will be acceptable."

He looked at me. He was about my height with brown hair and pale blue eyes that looked washed in bleach. He looked down at his shoes. "I'll see what I can do," he said. In a half hour he reported back that he'd found a bed. An ambulance was on its way. The ordeal had started at 9:30 that morning. The second ambulance arrived at 4:45 in the afternoon, and until that moment, I had completely forgotten about our dog, still in the back of my car at the doctor's office. I'd made arrangements for Tucker to go home from preschool with a friend, but I'd forgotten about Kodiak. Lee phoned our most resourceful friend, who drove over there and somehow managed to get him out of our locked car. We never did find out how.

While we waited for the ambulance to arrive, Lee pulled up a chair next to me and put his hands on top of mine on Andie's back. She was asleep. "Why now?" he asked. His eyes suddenly looked old. "We finally let our guard down." He rubbed his right eye and a stray lash fell on his cheek. "We finally opened our hearts—all the way." Tears slid down his face. "And look what happened."

The ambulance arrived to transfer us. The tall, older EMT looked at Andie asleep on my chest. "Looks like we're moving you two together," he said.

The bigger hospital was about 45 minutes away. But on a Friday night at rush hour it took a lot longer. Lee followed behind in his car. I lay in the back of the ambulance with Andie strapped to my chest. We inched along. I had to pee, but I didn't say a word. No jokes about quarts of milk this time. I had a job to do. I was breathing for my baby, and yes, I was scared, but I stayed present in my fear, refusing to let my baby go.

When we reached the hospital, Andie was placed in a quarantined RSV room. She was the only patient in a room with four beds. I thought about the ER doctor who'd told us no beds were available. We settled Andie in, and I climbed in beside her. The short, stocky nurse checking Andie's vitals looked down at me. "I'm sorry," she said. "You're going to have to get out of the bed."

I shook my head and said, "No."

She put her hand on her hip. "It's against hospital policy," she told me.

I stared out the window; it had gotten dark and the lights of the city were starting to come on. Time to use my new voice again. "I'm sleeping next to my baby," I said.

Lee watched this exchange, and tried to hide his smile. The nurse huffed out of the room, her rubber shoes squeaking as she went. She returned waving a form I had to sign, releasing the hospital of any liability if I fell out of the bed in the middle of the night.

When she left, Lee and I laughed. Then we sighed. It was

late. We were tired. "I should go get Tucker," Lee whispered,
reaching out to rub my arm. "I want to let him know Andie
will be okay."

I looked down at Andie curled up next to me, asleep.
"Don't go," I whispered back.

"I have to go, babe," he said.

I watched him. "I'm scared."

"Me too," he bent down and kissed Andie lightly on the
head. Then he kissed me. And then he walked out the door. I
was alone with my baby, breathing for her.

◆

Karen McCarthy came to the hospital the next day while
Tucker was cuddling with Andie in her bed. I met her at
the door. I didn't even say hello. "Why is this happening?" I
asked.

"Nice to see you, too." She smiled.

"Really," I said. "Why?"

Karen put her hands on my shoulders. "This is your second chance," she said. "A chance to get everything right that
you missed the first time."

I thought a moment, and then I nodded. I knew exactly
what she meant. I thought of Tucker, arriving that morning.
"Hi Andie," he'd said, climbing into bed next to her. "You
okay? Whatcha watchin'?" Leaning into each other, they
gazed up at the TV.

Before now, Tucker had been kept away from the hospital. This morning he was with his sister, right where he
belonged. We were getting it right.

And I was remaining present, being accountable and

staying responsible. The previous night I'd learned how to use a nebulizer and administer the breathing therapy Andie needed every two hours. When *I* taught *Lee* the next day his eyes crinkled in delight, noticing the role reversal.

We stood just inside the door as I listed all these achievements for Karen. "Good," she said, nodding her head. "Because as soon as Andie is well enough, get the hell out of here." She pointed across the hall. Through a door we could see nurses putting on masks, hospital gowns, and gloves to enter. We didn't know what was happening in that room. We didn't want to.

And just as quickly as Andie became sick, she seemed to recover. Before we were discharged we were given a nebulizer, albuterol, and inhalable steroids to take home. When Lee asked about possible side effects, the doctor said, "Well, over time, the steroids might inhibit her growth," as he scrawled on his prescription pad. When I looked up with wild eyes, he added, "Just an inch or two."

"Oh is that all?" I asked, and Lee put his hand on my shoulder and pulled me to him.

Two days (which felt like two months) later, we were on our way home. Lee drove slowly. I rested my head back against the seat, thinking how we'd dodged yet another bullet.

A squeaky sound came from the back. And for just a moment, I pretended not to hear. I was too exhausted to look. Besides, what else could possibly go wrong? But that maternal instinct nagged, and I turned.

There was Tucker, perched in his car seat with a plastic

sandwich bag stuck over his head. Every time he breathed, his mouth and nose sucked in the plastic.

I ripped the bag off his head. "Are you *fucking* kidding me?" I yelled at the roof of the car. "Enough," I shouted, hoping someone, somewhere might be listening. "We've had enough. *We are done.*"

26

Germs

✦

For two years, I'd been a diligent soldier in the fight against germ warfare; I'd done everything I could to keep Andie isolated from illness, so she would never have to fend off more than a mild cold. Every day when Tucker returned from preschool I'd stripped him down at the door. His schoolboy, germ-infested clothing went straight into the washer and his contaminated hands went straight to the sink. I was fanatic about it, and when we lost the battle against RSV, I got even more gung ho about keeping the house germ-free. While my hands grew red and chapped from washing, the stories I'd heard about my uncle's sister kept running through my mind.

My uncle's sister had obsessive-compulsive disorder (OCD). Her three children, who were about my age growing up, would arrive home from school and come in through the garage, where the washing machine was. They'd strip off every article of clothing and put them in the washer, and when they were naked, they'd proceed to the door, knock and wait. Rather than greeting them with cookies and milk, their mother came out with a big spray bottle of Lysol. After they were sprayed from top to bottom, they were permitted to enter.

The scary thing was, as I played the border guard in my own war against germs, I totally understood where that crazy lady was coming from. And ever since the RSV, as I conducted my own daily strip searches, I could feel my feet sliding down that slippery slope from normal toward completely off my rocker.

"Post-traumatic stress disorder?" I asked Dr. Shah. "I'm not a Vietnam vet." It had been two weeks since Andie had been released from the hospital, and I was in his office for my annual exam. "I'm a 34-year-old mom living in the suburbs of Boston." I picked up my purse from the chair next to the exam table.

"From everything I've read, Kate," Dr. Shah leaned against the counter. "It's very common for parents of a premature baby to experience post-traumatic stress. You've been through a lot."

"Oh," I said, slipping into my shoes. "I'm sure I'll be fine."

I didn't want to believe him, but Dr. Shah was right. No bombs were exploding in my head, but every day I grew more OCD and was haunted by the memory of those doctor's words: *These x-rays have me freaked . . . it's up to her.* The words chanted at me as I loomed over Andie's crib, watching her inhale and exhale each breath. Lying back in my bed, I listened for sounds of breathing distress coming from her room and wondered, *How could I not have known my own child was struggling to breathe?* and, *How will I know if it's happening again?*

When I took Andie for her check-up, I complained to the nurse that I hadn't been able to tell if she was having trouble breathing. "Oh the signs are obvious," the nurse said with a wave of her hand. I stared at the shiny linoleum floor. *Well, if that's the case, why hadn't I seen the signs a week before?*

"There are certain things to look for." She pulled up Andie's t-shirt without really looking at her. "See? That's normal breathing." She pointed to Andie's middle. "If she was struggling, her stomach would be pulling."

"*Pulling?*" I asked, moving closer to study Andie's little belly.

"Yeah. Her stomach would be pulling in under her ribs if she was struggling."

"Oh," I pretended I understood. At home I constantly lifted Andie's little cotton shirts to study her belly as she tried to break free. Was she pulling? I could never tell.

That nurse also told me I could time her number of breaths per minute. The second night Lee was away on his business trip to Colorado—a trip I would no longer even discuss going on—I called him in a panic at three in the morning. "I've been trying to time her breaths," I cried over the phone. "And I can't tell if she's okay." I pictured him lying in a hotel bed, holding his watch up to the light, measuring the seconds on his end of the phone while I counted her breaths on mine.

That week, my nursing friend, Stephanie, taught me how to listen to Andie's lungs with a stethoscope to ensure they were clear. A few days later, my friend, Nancy, from book group, came over and shared her secrets for surviving her daughter's asthma. She suggested I thumbtack a list of breathing distress symptoms to the back of my bathroom door so that, even in the heat of the moment, I could think clearly.

When the local fire chief (whose crew had transported Andie from the pediatric office to the hospital) called to see how she was doing, I confessed my fears about her lingering breathing issues. He told me to call anytime, day or night, and his rescue crew would come check her out.

I was making myself, and everyone else, crazy.

Finally, I called the nurse at the doctor's office and asked about buying an oximeter, the little machine used to measure Andie's breathing rate. "Forget it," she said. "They cost about a thousand bucks." But Lee found one online for three hundred.

That little machine was worth its weight in gold. All I had to do was stick Andie's index finger into the bright yellow square, about the size of a ring box. Within seconds, a flashing red light displayed her blood/oxygen level. The oximeter was certain; I didn't have to rely on my own uncertain assessment. I could hold it in the palm of my hand, and it would confirm that my daughter was okay.

27

Glasses

✦

THAT SAME WINTER, Andie's early intervention coordinator expressed concerns that she wasn't using as
many words as a "normal" two-year-old. Terry, a speech and
language therapist, started coming on Tuesday mornings to
work with Andie.

In the meantime, Karen McCarthy recommended we
enroll Andie in a music class. "You should also work with
a cranial-sacral therapist," she said. "What's cranial-sacral
therapy?" I asked, balancing the phone on my shoulder and
spooning macaroni and cheese onto the kids' dinner plates.
"Cranial-sacral therapy uses light touch to work on the
body's craniosacral system—the bones, nerves, and connec-
tive tissues of the cranium and spine," she told me. "Some
practitioners do myofascial release as well, which focuses on
restrictions within the fascia tissue, the tissue between the
skin and muscle. If you pull back the skin of a chicken, that
white stringy stuff is the fascia." *Eeew,* I thought. "Babs, the
woman I recommend, is fantastic and works a lot with kids.
Give her a call."

✦

Babs greeted us at the door of her office, wearing mascu-
line clothing and thick glasses. She was short and stout, but

sturdy, and right away she asked us to remove our shoes. I smiled.

"She's not talking, then?" she asked as I helped Andie out of her coat.

"Not much." I watched Babs put a pegboard and colorful pegs on the blue gymnastics mat on the floor. Andie went right over. I stood just inside the door in my socks.

"What does she call you and your husband?" Babs asked.

"Mom and Dad."

"Huh." She sat down cross-legged on the floor behind Andie, who was busy sticking pegs on the board and hardly noticed when Babs gently placed her hands on her back and head. I sat down on the edge of a chair against the wall.

"And she has an older brother?"

"Yup. Tucker." I said. "Two years older."

We sat in silence for several minutes while Babs moved her hands up and down Andie's back. A mobile of origami birds hanging from the ceiling slowly turned in the breeze from an open window.

Toward the end of the appointment, Babs turned and looked at me. She kept her hands on Andie's back. "This girl can talk," she said. "She's got plenty of words in her. She's just *choosing* not to use them."

I remembered Lee's mom telling me over Thanksgiving that Andie had walked up to her with a video in hand and said, "I wanna watch this." I'd dismissed it at the time, thinking there was no way Andie could have actually spoken all those words.

Babs put her hands on Andie's neck and tilted her head. She watched Andie playing with the pegs. I liked Babs. I felt somehow comforted in her office with the blue mats and the children's pictures on the wall. "Andie and Tucker are communicating telepathically," she said, dropping her hands to Andie's shoulders. "They're speaking with their minds. And as long as he reads her thoughts and acts as her spokesperson," Babs shrugged and looked at Andie, "her needs are met. She doesn't need language." I sat back in the chair and nodded. I knew what she was talking about. Lee and I were guilty, too. We always seemed to know what she needed without her asking.

Babs smiled. "Don't read her mind," she said. "Let her say what she needs."

On the drive home, I glanced at Andie in the rearview mirror, kicking her feet in her car seat and twirling her hair with her finger. Andie will start talking, I decided. We'd stop doing it for her. I read somewhere that if you want kids to overcome frustration, you have to let them get frustrated. If you want them to pick themselves up, you have to let them fall down. And if you want them to talk, I added, looking back at Andie's big hazel eyes watching the world go by out the window, *you gotta stop talking for them.*

That afternoon when Tucker was playing in the sandbox, I called him over and held his hands in mine. "Tuck?"

"Yeah?" His lashes were so long they made shadows on his cheeks.

"You want Andie to talk, right?"

He nodded. He was wearing his Superman shirt, and he looked very brave, holding my fingers in his hand.

"So you know how you listen to her thoughts and speak for her?"

He nodded.

"Well, now we have to try to not do that anymore. We have to let her talk instead. Do you understand that?"

He yawned. "Okay," he said and then he ran off across the backyard on his little legs.

A few days later, the kids and I were sitting at the kitchen table eating lunch. Tuck's peanut butter and jelly sandwich was cut into four squares, and he had jam on his cheeks. Andie sat in her booster seat, staring at her empty plate.

"Andie," I said, holding up my props. "Which one do you want, the apple or the banana?"

She stared at me and blinked her big eyes.

"Apple or banana," I said louder.

Nothing.

"Come on, Andie," I tried again, "Which do you want, the apple or the banana?"

Tucker looked up, grabbed the banana and handed it to Andie. "The banana," he said. "She wants the banana."

So much for my plan of letting Andie talk for herself.

✦

Then we discovered it wasn't only her speech. One morning after visiting Babs, I was sitting at the kitchen table next to Andie as she drew on paper. "What are you drawing?" I asked.

She kept scribbling on her paper with her red crayon. "Tucker."

"Tucker's a handsome big brother," I picked up a crayon to doodle on the edge of the paper. Andie went back to her drawing, but this time I noticed she tilted her head and moved it down toward the paper. Her little pink tongue poked out from the side of her mouth. Her left eye was only a couple inches away from her drawing.

I scheduled an appointment with Dr. V., her eye surgeon, and to everyone's surprise (including Dr. V.'s), Andie was straining to see well out of her non-surgical eye.

"She's gonna need glasses," Dr. V. said, sliding her stool back from her desk. I frowned as she handed me the eyeglass prescription. I didn't want my two-year-old to need glasses.

"There's nothing cuter than a little girl in glasses," my dad said over the phone.

"I'm worried she'll feel different," I said

"She's lucky," Tucker piped up from the spot on the kitchen rug where he was lining up his trucks. I hadn't known he was listening, and an idea popped into my head: Andie could get prescription glasses, while Tucker would get glasses with clear lenses. I whispered my thought into the phone. "Sounds like a clever plan, Arnold," my dad said.

The next day, we headed off to Target optical and Richard, a tall, dark man with a beautiful Caribbean accent, found a little pink pair that fit Andie's thin face perfectly. Tucker picked out a pair of round frames, and when he turned around from the mirror, he had a big grin on his face. "A blond Harry Potter," Richard said.

We were all happy as we strolled over to the register to pay. Mission accomplished. Richard punched a bunch of numbers in the computer and announced the total. I stared at the number. How could it be so much? On the way out, I studied the receipt. Tucker's fake glasses had cost 20 bucks more than Andie's real ones! But for the next two weeks, he wore them to school and received lots of compliments from his teachers and classmates. He would soon abandon them, but Andie would wear hers every moment of the day, taking them off only for bed and bath.

✦

Karen McCarthy introduced me to a series of fun eye exercises that I could play with the kids to help improve Andie's vision. I taped a series of different-colored electrical tape on either end of a dowel rod and Andie held the rod out in front of her with both hands. I'd cover one of her eyes with a "pirate patch" and call out a color. Andie would try and hit the wiffle ball I'd hung from the ceiling with the matching color on the stick. Then we'd switch the patch to the other eye and play again.

In another exercise, Lee made a balance beam with a leftover two-by-four. With one eye patched, the kids would walk backwards and forwards on the beam, catching beanbags and dropping them into buckets along the way.

The games were meant for Andie, but Tucker loved them, too. One early intervention specialist dubbed him Andie's best physical therapist because she'd do anything to keep up with him. Out in the backyard Tuck would yell, "Race ya, Andie!" In her orange dress and little pink high tops she'd chase him to the swing set where he'd yell, "I win!" and Andie, following close behind, would call out, "I looooose!"

I heard it said that the eyes are the windows to the soul. There had been times during the past two years when I'd looked into the depth of Andie's eyes and thought I'd caught glimpses of ancient worlds, lifetimes of history. But now, looking at her eyes through the lenses of her glasses, I saw muscles that could be exercised and strengthened.

We focused on strengthening her other muscles, too. Lee hung a set of gymnastics rings between two trees and a horse swing from the swing set, both excellent for strengthening core muscles. A friend loaned us an old-fashioned rocking horse and the kids rode that in our living room like cowboys on a wild bucking bronco.

An amazing thing happened when those glasses went on Andie's face. All her stored-up words began tumbling out. The floodgates opened. Not just a few words here and there, but streams of words strung together in recognizable phrases. "I want cookie," she'd say or "More juice, Mommy please," or "No, not go to bed." It was incredible. There was obviously a connection between her sight and her speech. I'd later meet a special needs teacher who shared several stories of students whose language dramatically improved once an eye impairment was discovered.

So between the cranial-sacral therapy, the work with the early intervention specialists, and Andie's new glasses, we were on our way to that day when I'd happily complain, "Will this girl ever stop talking?"

28

Changes

♦

ANDIE WAS DOING WELL, but the trauma of RSV had not left us. I was still so afraid we'd lose her. It seemed like she was sick all the time, and with every cold her lungs struggled. She'd have to inhale a steroid twice a day and the lung-expanding drug, albuterol, every four hours, even in the middle of the night. Lee rigged a system where her teddy bear "held" the mouthpiece of the nebulizer to her face so we could doze nearby on the floor.

We began calling these ordinary colds that left her struggling to breathe, "RSV echoes." Our doctor hadn't used the term asthma, but it was becoming clear that's where we were headed. It was a chicken-and-egg scenario. Did the RSV lead to the asthma, or had her lungs always been this vulnerable?

I made an appointment with a pulmonologist at Children's Hospital and listened to the petite doctor with tight curls tell me that because of her birth history, Andie would never be cured of asthma. I declined her offer to prescribe a variety of daily preventative drugs. Instead, I tried to strengthen Andie's lungs my own way. At a physical therapy supply store, I bought a bunch of "lung development games" and brought home straws, feathers, and cotton balls, cheering the kids on as they blew the "bunny tails" across the kitchen table. The kids and I blew up balloons and played kazoos, harmonicas, and whistles.

Lee had his own "Daddy Lung Improvement Program." Every night when he walked through the back door, the kids ran to him, wrapping their arms and legs around him. "Tickle monster, tickle monster, Daddy!" They'd scream, and Lee would hold his arms out in the air, curl his fingers, and growl as the kids ran, screaming, into the living room. There they'd all fall in a tickling heap. Between her screams, Andie would howl with laughter and gulp in big breaths of air. Just when it seemed she couldn't take it any more, she'd call out, "Tickle me more, Daddy!"

Lee was also convinced that good, old-fashioned winter air was some of the best lung medicine available. Like the asthma medicine, the cold air caused the lungs to expand. We bundled Andie up in warm thermal layers and out she'd go. She was on her first pair of skis at age two.

From Karen McCarthy I learned that the lungs, skin, and gut are all closely connected. Asthma sufferers, she explained, often have skin issues or intestinal problems or both. Traditional medicine compartmentalizes the body, looking at each part—the lungs, heart, skin, intestines and brain—separately and then trying to put them together like pieces of a jigsaw puzzle. But the body doesn't work that way. Nothing works independently. Karen taught us that holistic medicine looks at the whole body, and sees that every part is connected. Since the gut was at the heart of a well-functioning body, if we wanted Andie's lungs to strengthen, we needed to focus on improving the health of her gut. I approached this from a dietary stand-point, recognizing that what went in (and what came out) was vital to her health.

As our diets and awareness changed, I started reading la-bels and noticing that additives, preservatives, and dyes were in a lot of the foods we ate. In the cafeteria line in fifth grade, I remembered hearing that the dye in red Jell-O caused can-cer, but I'd never thought about it beyond that. I learned from Karen that our livers become overtaxed by trying to get rid of all those harmful toxins. And with the liver over-taxed, the kidneys start working harder and become flood-ed, which leads to more toxins building up in the system. I worked at keeping the kids' kidneys warm and dry. Once out of the bath, I'd blow dry their lower backs and massage their kidneys. Whenever Andie had a cold, she rested on a heating pad so we could dry out and support her kidneys.

Every morning, I'd put supplements in either a smooth-ie or a bowl of oatmeal, fortifying her gut with a probiotic (good bacteria that aid in the production of flora in the in-testinal tract) and essential fatty acids like flaxseed and bor-age oils. The kids learned the importance of pooping, the body's everyday way of cleaning out any leftover "junk." "I just pooped!" they'd exclaim to cheers of "hooray!" If con-stipation became an issue, we used George's Aloe Vera Juice, which is clear and tasteless and anyone who has tried it can vouch for how fast it works.

I also found an anti-inflammatory herb called mullein and made tea for Andie when her lungs were acting up. The tea had remarkably positive results. I put in lots of locally harvested honey, which helped build up her immune system to the environmental allergens in our region.

I learned a whole, healthy body needs a strong immune system. If the lymph glands are bogged down because they're trying to rid the body of toxins, they don't have the strength to do the real job of keeping the body healthy. Karen taught me how to give lymphatic massage to drain the system, and every day the kids jumped on a mini-trampoline to keep their lymphatic systems active.

My yoga teacher, Nancy, taught Andie how to breathe deeply by placing a stuffed animal on her belly and teaching her to use her breath to make it rise and fall. She also gave us a recipe for an anti-viral room spray that contained essential oils like clove, cinnamon, and thyme. I don't know if it worked, but our house always smelled delicious. Once aware of how hard our bodies had to work just to process the pollution in the air we breathe, I started making natural cleaning products with vinegar and lavender oil.

All of Andie's traditional medical doctors were—and continue to be—an invaluable part of her journey, but this holistic approach made so much sense to me. To the benefit of all of us, we managed to find just the right balance between these two worlds. I would often say that traditional medicine kept Andie alive, and holistic medicine allowed her to thrive.

I was empowering myself and taking control of our lives. By actively doing something about our circumstances, I was no longer playing the role of a victim. The puzzle pieces of my life were slowly starting to come together. As I worked on healing my daughter, I was beginning to heal myself.

29

Ghosts

+

WHEN ANDIE TURNED THREE, testing determined she was on par with children her own age and she "graduated" from Children's Hospital's infant follow-up program with flying colors. When we left the hospital, Andie carried her very own diploma with her name printed boldly across the top in black marker. Margaret, her early intervention service coordinator, brought a vanilla cupcake with colored sprinkles to the house on her very last visit. She put her arm around Andie while I took their photo.

One morning, not long afterward, Lee and I awoke and pulled ourselves up until our heads met on the pillow. "Hi," he whispered. "Hi," I whispered back. The kids had climbed in with us sometime in the early morning hours and were sleeping soundly beneath our covers. "You look cute in the morning," Lee said. I snuggled in closer to him. He looked down at the kids and said, "Andie's hair's getting longer." Her butter-colored hair fanned out around her head like a halo. "I keep having this vision," he said, sliding his arm in back of me so I could rest my head more easily on his shoulder, "She's skiing down the slopes, with her long hair flying behind her."

I kissed him on the cheek and thought about how slowly Andie's hair grew. It had taken so long until it finally grew past her ears and no longer needed a barrette to hold it back. I remembered the nights Lee sat on the edge of her bed, brushing her hair.

One day, just after Andie turned three, she walked into the kitchen holding hands with Lee. "Show Mommy," he said. Andie had turned around to show me her short, bouncy ponytail.

And not long after, Lee was away on a business trip and I had to call him and report that Tucker had cut Andie's hair.

My mom had gone away that same week to a spa with girlfriends, so rather than fly solo and stay home by himself, my dad came down to help with the kids.

"Where are you going, Mommy?" Andie asked as she and Tucker jumped on the living room couch.

"I'm going to get my haircut." I kissed both of them on their little foreheads. "Papa Jer's gonna watch you until I get back." I practically bounced across the driveway to my car, happy to have a few hours to myself so I could be pampered at the salon.

A few hours later, I walked in the back door, my freshly cut hair swinging against my back. Dad was at the kitchen table with the phone pressed to his ear and a bunch of papers spread out before him. He pointed to my hair, smiled, and gave me a thumbs up. "Where are the kids?" I mouthed. He pointed up.

"Hey guys," I called from the bottom of the stairs. "Mommy's home." I heard a little giggle. "Are you guys hiding?" I started up the stairs, and when I got to the hallway, I heard a rustling behind Tuck's closed door. "I know where you are," I called, as I pushed opened his door.

Andie was sitting crossed-legged on the edge of Tuck's bed, and Tucker was at her side with a dull pair of school scissors in his hand.

"Hi Mom," Tuck grinned.

"Hey, bud," I said. "What are you guys up—?" And then I noticed the long strands of blond hair covering the front of Andie's black turtleneck. A pair of short jagged bangs ran across her forehead and random long and short pieces hung on either side. I put my hands over my eyes. "Noooo," I moaned.

"It was me!" Tucker said in his proud five-year-old voice. "I cut Andie's hair! Now it won't get in her eyes anymore!"

My mouth opened and closed but no words came out.

Turning around, I ran into the hall, leaned over the stairs and screamed, "Daaaaad!"

As we assessed the damage to Andie's hair, Dad kept patting my back and saying "Two minutes, I was on the phone for two minutes. I could already hear him re-telling the story at next weekend's cocktail parties. He looked at Tucker. "How could you do this to Papa Jer, Tucker?"

I pulled Tucker into my lap. "You're the one who left them alone," I said.

◆

It took a year for the damage from Tucker's Beauty School to grow out. One morning, I was playing with Andie's newly grown-out hair while she was lying on the floor, playing dollhouse. I watched her carefully put the dog outside, Mom in the kitchen and Dad in the living room. She put the little girl on the bed in the upstairs bedroom.

"Is the little girl going to sleep?" I asked, tucking a loose strand of her hair behind her ear.

"Yeah," Andie said. "And then the man behind her bed will say 'Boo' and wake her up."

My skin went cold. Andie woke up almost every night in the middle of the night and one of us would have to rock her back to sleep. I watched her move the tiny furniture around the miniature rooms. "What man?" I asked.

"The man in my room," Andie said.

Too stunned to ask any more questions, my mind raced around for an explanation. I thought back to the first night Lee and I had slept in our new 200-year-old house. We'd curled up on a futon in front of the fireplace in the upstairs bedroom and at three in the morning I'd woken with a start. Someone, *something* was holding my hand. I snatched it back. My scream woke Lee. We lay breathing in the dark; both agreeing it must have been my imagination.

In the same room, three years later, I was lying on my side resting with newborn Tucker when I felt a gentle hug from behind. Still half-asleep, I thought, *Mmm, that's sweet, Lee's lying down with us.* Then my mind snapped awake, and I remembered Lee was at work. I flipped on my back, my heart pounding and my eyes wide open.

While I watched Andie earnestly moving the dollhouse people around, I thought about those nights when I'd been nursing Tucker and I'd sometimes see a swirling purplish light on the otherwise dark ceiling. When I told Lee, he thought I was crazy until one night I whispered in his ear, "Lee, wake up." He moaned awake and flipped on his back.

"Look. Do you see it?" He put his head next to mine on my pillow. "Yes," he whispered. "I do see it." Then he rolled over and went back to sleep.

When Tucker was one, I met a woman at a friend's engagement party who mentioned she was psychic and knew about spirits. How *that* came up in conversation I can't remember, but I do remember telling her what was happening at our house.

Her eyes got big, and she leaned in closer to me. "Do you have any animals?" she'd asked.

"Yeah, a dog and a cat." She'd stared at me so intently, I looked down at my drink.

"Do they go in the room?" she'd asked.

I thought about it and realized that we couldn't drag Kodi over the threshold. Our cat, Seal? I couldn't recall ever seeing him in that room. "No, they don't go in the room."

"That confirms it." She rocked up on her toes. "You've got a spirit all right." She took a sip of her drink. "Probably feels its job is to protect you. But still, you gotta ask it to go."

So following her instructions, I sprinkled salt in each corner of the room, lit a white candle, and said, "You can go now. Please, leave," in a quiet, shaky voice. I was worried a neighbor might walk by and see me through the window, but I said it again, louder this time, "Go, please. You're free to leave now."

That seemed to do it. We didn't have any more encounters and for several years we lived in ghost-free peace until the dollhouse incident.

As soon as Andie was asleep on the couch that afternoon,

I marched into her room, not bothering with the salt and white candle, and simply demanded whomever, whatever was bothering my daughter, to get the hell out of our house. "This child needs all the sleep she can get." I shook my clenched fists in the air. "How dare you wake her up at night? Leave at once." I pointed to the window I'd just opened, thinking it might give the spirit an easy escape route.

A few days later, Lee and I were lying in bed when our bedroom door flew open, and Andie walked in. I gasped. Her beautiful blond hair was hacked into a jagged, horrible mess. Walking right over to my side of the bed, she ceremoniously delivered her shorn locks in a velvet purse from her dress-up box.

Tucker had cut her a set of bangs. But this time, Andie had managed to create the worst-looking haircut in history; nearly scalping her left side, cutting a crooked line across her forehead, and shearing the crown so her hair stuck up like a baby chick. She'd left the back long, like a 1980s' rock star.

My mom came two days later, and as we walked Andie toward her preschool door, she doubled over, laughing so hard that she had to wipe the tears from her eyes. "What's so funny?" I asked.

She pointed to a sign posted on the door. "TODAY IS PIC-TURE DAY!"

I laughed right along with her, but it kept bothering me that Andie had delivered her slashed-off hair like a gift. Lee said it was because we were stupid enough to let her keep scissors in her room. I thought something else might be going on. While I was taking Andie's hat off that evening,

I touched her hacked-up hair and thought, *Have I declared war with a ghost?* As if reading my thoughts, Lee said, "Kasey, we left scissors in her room. There's nothing more to it." But I wasn't convinced. I thought it was time to bring in an expert.

She called herself a "house healer" and arrived with two colleagues and an Alaskan Malamute. Her cheeks were apple red and her gray bobbed hair swung side to side when she walked. I looked down at her playful eyes and noted how warm her hand felt when we shook.

She and her team of two others spent the next two hours going through the house. We weren't sure exactly what they were doing. They began in the basement and ended in the attic. Occasionally, one of them called out or moaned loudly and the dog barked twice. As instructed, we sat on the kitchen barstools with a white candle lit for our protection and talked in whispers, glancing at the clock above the stove.

We knew the clearing was over when "the team" walked into the kitchen all smiles. Even the dog seemed to be smiling. The leader stepped forward and walked over to the kitchen island. "Well." She placed her palms flat on the butcher block. "You had a lot going on." She cleared her throat. "I'm not surprised, given the age of the house and all, but even the newer houses have plenty of unwanted energies left over from previous owners, living or dead." She smiled back at her team. Apparently that was an inside joke. "Anyway, we've got a lot of historical information about the house if you're interested."

Lee pushed his stool back and stood up slowly. "You know what," he said, "part of me is really curious, but the other part worries . . ." Instead of finishing, he looked over at me and put his hand on my shoulder. "I think it's just as well if we don't know."

So the house healers left and we stood alone in the kitchen, looking at each other.

"Do you feel it?" Lee looked up at the ceiling. "I mean, hear it?"

"What?" I asked.

"The quiet . . . the lack of noise. There was always a kind of humming sound. It's gone."

The house felt still, almost silent. "Yeah," I said. "I do."

Lee went off to work, and that afternoon a colleague walked into the coffee room as Lee was filling his mug.

"You in late this morning?" he asked.

"Yeah," Lee said.

"Doctor's appointment?" his friend asked.

"No," Lee said. "Ghostbusters."

✦

In the weeks following the clearing, I started to notice subtle changes in our lives. Kodi and Seal were suddenly in and out of Tucker and Andie's rooms all the time, but more important, the constant feeling of chaos and disorganization in our house wasn't there anymore. Everything felt clearer, more ordered. It was like we'd stopped moving in circles and finally found our path forward.

Friends teased us about our "haunted house." My family thought I'd fallen off the deep end. I didn't care. I was willing to do anything and everything to keep our family safe. Who knows? If a house can be healed, why not the folks inside, too?

30

Moments

✦

W INTER WAS JUST AROUND the corner. We were
worried about another season of recurrent illnesses
and feeling a little hopeless about keeping Andie healthy. Until one day Karen McCarthy asked, "Why don't you just keep
Tucker out of school for the winter? A winter without sickness might give Andie's lungs time to heal and strengthen."

So after long debates and discussions with Tucker's
teachers, Andie's pediatrician, and each other, we decided to
keep Tucker home.

We'd just moved him to a new full-day preschool program where he seemed to adjust easily, and I felt guilty (as I
did about everything) taking him away from his pre-school
friends and his routine, but we knew it was the right thing
to do. He finished the last day before Christmas vacation and
wouldn't go back until April.

I wondered what I'd do with the kids for three months
during winter. I couldn't take them to indoor (germ-infested) museums, libraries, and gymnastic centers. It would defeat the whole purpose of keeping Tucker home. So instead, I
bundled them up and we went to deserted beaches, outdoor
zoos, and empty playgrounds. We did arts and crafts projects
on the dining room table and read lots of books by the fire.

It ended up being a marvelous winter. Without a prescribed agenda, our days were slow and calm. It was like an out-of-season summer vacation.

When the crocuses and daffodils emerged, so did we. Andie had been kept healthy and Tucker trotted back to his preschool classroom. But his teachers reported he was struggling to find a place in the class after such a long absence. I understood, because I was having trouble fitting in again, too. I'd always been a bit of a loner, but that winter I had really withdrawn, and now I wanted to keep turning inward as a threesome, shutting out the rest of the world. It took a lot of effort just to carry on everyday conversations.

At Coffee Haven, the little café at the end of our street where local artists hung their colorful paintings, Andie and I would sit at a corner table. I drank coffee, while she sipped her hot cocoa and ate a bagel with cream cheese. Around us, groups of moms and kids sat in noisy bunches. I overheard bits of conversations about celebrities, TV shows, and upcoming parties in town. Their conversations felt shallow, pointless. I wanted to talk about homeopathy, lymphatic massage, and how it feels to think your child is going to die. I knew I didn't fit in, but just in case they thought I might, I built an invisible wall around myself, making me even more unapproachable.

Spring and summer passed in this way.

Then fall arrived. It was time for Tuck to start kindergarten. Lee took the morning off from work, and we all walked him to school for his first big day. I didn't cry until Tucker brushed Andie's grown-out hair off her shoulders and kissed her on the cheek. "Bye, Andie," he said and then he turned to walk into the classroom, his Spiderman backpack bouncing on his shoulders.

A few days later, we drove Andie to Full Circle Farm, where she'd be going to preschool two mornings every week. In the yard some kids were already playing. Not far away, a few sheep were grazing. Lois, her teacher, rolled up the sleeves on her denim shirt, squatted down, and shook Andie's hand. "I'm glad you're here, Andie," she said. Andie smiled and slowly began walking toward the swings. Lois turned to me. "How are you doing, Mom?"

"Ah . . ." I said, watching Andie talking to a little girl in brown braids. "This is hard. Scary for me."

She patted my back. "We'll keep her safe. Remember, I'm Lois the clean freak. I'll send a kid home if he comes in with so much as a runny nose."

I let out a big breath. "Thanks, Lois," I said. "That's why she's here."

As the year progressed, I withdrew further into myself. I took long walks and started going to the coffee shop in the next town over, where I didn't know anyone. I was lonely, but I wanted to be alone. Andie, on the other hand, was a budding social butterfly. She'd bop up to me on the play yard when I came to pick her up, her blond ponytail swinging. "Mommy, mommy," she'd cry, her warm little fingers gripping mine. "I want Ashley to come over. Can you ask her mom?" And then she'd pull me toward a mother holding a bunch of papers, a pocketbook, a child's jacket, and an awkward clay sculpture that looked about to lose its parts. "Mrs.

Wells, this is my mom!" Andie would say, holding her other hand out to a little red-haired girl and smiling happily. "Can Ashley come to our house?" In that way, I was forced to introduce myself to other moms and make proper arrangements.

At our sessions, Karen McCarthy talked a great deal about my inability to stay present. She leaned forward in her office chair and touched my knee. "You're always checking out," she said. "Try staying present and really be in the moment. When you're with your kids, *be* with them. And be present not just with them, but all the time. In the grocery store, really look at the fruits and vegetables. Appreciate the colors. On your walks, notice the trees, feel the wind on your cheeks. Be in the moment."

By the end of that appointment we came up with the technique of asking myself *Am I present?* several times a day. It actually helped. During the morning drop-off at Andie's school I talked more with other parents and even arranged a few playdates without Andie's prodding. I felt more comfortable inside my own skin.

Then I had what I've come to call my "shopping cart moment." It was one of those mornings when I raced the kids to school, then zoomed off to try to do way more errands than time could possibly allow. I was zipping through the grocery store, throwing things in my cart, thinking about my next stop, and checking my watch when the question rang in my mind. *Kasey, are you present?* I laughed out loud. A big woman in a red hat turned around and frowned at me. I looked down at my shoes. "No," I whispered to the shopping cart. I took a deep breath, pulled out my to-do list, and scratched off all the other errands. I decided that while I filled my grocery cart, I would stay fully present and enjoy the experience. In the produce section, I studied the bright red tomatoes, smelled the strawberries, and rubbed the melons. I wandered around and found foods I never even knew the store carried. I was delighted when recipe ideas popped into my head.

Eventually, I arrived at the checkout. The lines were several customers deep. I wanted to fret, but instead I took my spot as third in line and waited. Soon more shoppers were waiting behind me. *Yes,* I boasted out loud in my head, *I am present.*

The line moved, and I was up next.

Preparing to unload my cart, I looked down. Then I looked down again. I looked behind me, then back into the cart.

It was empty. My shopping cart was empty. I'd stood in line for ten minutes clinging to the handle of an empty shopping cart.

Later I'd laugh when I told Lee, but in the meantime I had to excuse myself, reverse my empty cart under the scrutiny of the other shoppers, and find my way back *out* of line.

"I forgot something," I muttered as I walked past the staring customers.

Yeah, your mind, their looks seemed to say.

I searched several aisles and finally found my full cart waiting patiently alongside the canned tomatoes and imported olive oils. I must have walked away with an empty one that had been sitting near mine.

I swapped carts, and as I pushed my loaded cart back down the aisle I said out loud, *Kasey, are you present?* That time I refused to answer and went to find my place in line.

✦

So I was getting better at staying present, but I still had moments of checking out. One morning in June, I stood alongside the other mothers in the music teacher, Miss Diana's, house, waiting for Andie's music performance to begin. We could hear the children's voices from behind the closed door. A clock ticked on the mantel. Nearly every surface in the room was covered in lace doilies and china teacups. My friend Karen turned to me. "Kasey, do you know everyone here?" I shook my head. "Kasey is Andie's mom," she said to the others with her big smile. They nodded and began asking questions. "Where in town do you live?" "Do you have other children?" "Where does Andie go to school?" And then one of them asked me, "When is Andie's birthday?"

"November," I said. "The twenty-seventh."

"How old will she be?" she asked.

I stared back at the woman, who was smiling expectantly. I thought and thought, but my mind was completely blank. My silence drew everyone's attention. I knew Andie's birthday was in November, and I knew Andie was four, but my logic stopped there. It was like a big, black curtain had been pulled across my brain. I knew there was another number after four, but I just couldn't see it.

Karen stepped to my side and put her arm around me. "Five," she said. "She'll turn five in November."

I looked at Karen. "What?" my voice sounded far away, as though I were talking from a great distance. "She'll be five?" I asked. *"Five years old?"*

The other moms backed away, and Karen laughed, trying to lessen their suspicions of drug abuse. "It's a long story," she said. And then, thankfully, the door opened and Miss Diana called us in for the performance.

As the children sang their sweet songs, I sat crossed-legged on Miss Diana's living room floor and stared at Andie. *Five? She was going to be five? How did that happen?*

I watched her pay close attention to Miss Diana's directions, tapping her tambourine, singing the notes, and spinning in a circle, all at the proper times.

Suddenly I saw clearly the amazing child before me. She was the vision I had held all those years ago, just after she was born. *I either see a funeral in a week or a beautiful, healthy five-year-old girl.*

My vision had become real. She was a healthy, living, breathing, real-life little girl. She was everything I'd ever hoped for. And I'd finally woken up enough to see it. At that moment I could say with certainty, *Yes, I am present.*

3 1

Stirrings

◆

IN THE FALL OF 2006, Tucker began second grade and
Andie started kindergarten. I knew I should probably feel
like crying, but as I watched her walking into the brightly
lit classroom with her ponytail bouncing on that blue Hello
Kitty backpack, I was too happy to cry. She turned back only
once, to wave. Our baby was officially off to school. And she
was one of the tallest kids in the class.

Each morning, we walked or rode our bikes to school.
I'd wave goodbye to them from the school door, a part of
me feeling sad, knowing I wouldn't see them again until I
picked them up at 3:00 P.M. Another part of me wanted to
kick my heels together and scream, "Yahoo!" It was the first
time since Tucker was born eight years before that I'd had
any significant time to myself.

I didn't make plans. I didn't think about what I'd do with
my days. Most days, I just kept going, walking or biking alone
for an hour or two. I'd breathe and think, or not think at all.
Sometimes I looked at the changing leaves and found myself
crying, remembering all we'd been through. Other times
I'd bubble up with gratitude for all our blessings. At home
I made myself tea and played music. I folded laundry, orga-
nized closets, and curled up on the couch to read. Whatever

I did, I took it slowly. Finally, there was no ticking clock in the background telling me *Hurry! Hurry!*

Then in October, a company in New Hampshire approached Lee about a job opening. He'd been in Boston with the same company for 15 years and had no intention of leaving. "But what the heck," he told me one night while I was rinsing the dishes, and he was putting them in the dishwasher. "Why not check it out?"

One interview led to the next and sure enough he ended up taking the job in New Hampshire. It was by no means an easy decision. I have the long pros and cons lists to prove it. Location should have been the biggest item on the list, but we decided that was essentially a wash. What was the difference between driving 24 miles into Boston, which took an hour, or driving 63 miles north to the Granite State, which also took an hour? Overall, the pros outweighed the cons and off he went, north instead of east.

After less than a week on the new job, he walked through the back door one night and said, "We gotta talk."

My stomach tightened. "Did you lose your job?" I put my hands over my eyes, afraid to look at him.

"No," he laughed. "I didn't lose my job." He peeled my hands off my face and pulled me in for a hug. "But I am gonna lose my mind," he said into my hair. "The commute is killing me."

I rubbed his back. "You'll get used to it, babe."

"That's the thing." He pulled back to look at me. "I don't know if I will." I watched him rub his forehead.

"Here." I opened the fridge and grabbed him a beer.

After he popped the cap off and took a long sip, he set the bottle down and looked at me. "I was kind of thinking that maybe . . ." his eyes crinkled in that way they did when he was about to ask for something that might bring on an onslaught, "we should think about moving."

"Moving?" I slapped my hand down on the counter. "Are you out of your mind? That wasn't part of the plan."

"I'm just asking you to *think* about it." He reached for my hand. I tried to pull away, but he pulled me closer. "Just give it a little thought." He kissed my ear. "That's all I'm asking."

So I did. I thought about it that night in my comfy bed. I thought about it the next morning while I was making breakfast in my sunny kitchen. I thought about it while I walked the kids to school through the neighborhood I adored. I thought about it when I watched the kids on the playground, surrounded by their friends. I thought about it when the sweet man at the five-and-dime snuck a chocolate in my purse. I thought about it when dear old Al waved goodbye at the hardware store. I thought about it arriving home from school at our farmhouse that we'd poured our hearts and souls into for 12 years. And I thought about it after school when the kids ran across the street to play with their friends who were like cousins to them.

That night, I met Lee at the back door. He looked pale and tired. I told him I'd thought about moving, and gave him all the reasons why my answer was "no." "We've spent over a decade renovating this house, and it's *finally finished*. The kids can *walk* to school. They have *tons* of friends. We *love* our friends and neighbors and *this* town." I kissed him on the cheek. "So I definitely thought about it, babe." I walked over to the stove where the pasta was boiling. "And there's no way I'm moving."

Lee pulled out a stool and sat down. He rubbed his eyes. "What about my commute?" He unbuttoned his shirt cuffs. "Did you factor that in?"

I stopped stirring the pasta and looked at him. I had to admit; I hadn't given his circumstances one moment of thought. "Sometimes you must think it's all about me," I said.

He laughed. "We're all like that." He loosened his tie.

By the end of the night we'd settled on a compromise: If we found a great school for the kids and another old house we loved, I would agree to move. I snuggled into my bed, convinced the chances were so slim that life as I knew it would never be at risk.

The following weekend we laid out a well-worn map of New Hampshire on the kitchen table. Lee pointed out all the ski areas we'd been to. In crayon, he drew a red circle around the towns that were a half hour from his office. Then we kissed the kids goodbye, told the sitter we'd be back late in the afternoon, and walked through the back door. My fingers lightly touched the door frame. *The door frame Lee built*, I thought.

No, I didn't want to move, but walking through that door I felt a subtle stirring of possibility. Is this a new beginning? Is this part of our journey with Andie, a fresh start where she's no longer the miracle baby, born too early? I couldn't help but wonder.

On the way out of town, we stopped for coffee. As we

put our cardboard cups in the car's cup holders, Lee turned to me. "Thanks for doing this," he said.

I touched his cheek. "If this is what it takes to spend a day alone with you, I'm in." Lee shook his head and smiled. I popped some road tunes in, and we headed north, out of town.

By the time we got to New Hampshire, I needed a nap. "Are you kidding me?" I said to him. "This drive takes *forever*."

He nodded. "Try it at rush hour," he said.

"And then you have to do it again at the end of the day?" I patted his leg. "That's too much."

Lee turned left off the exit onto Route 101A. "Let's go take a look at some towns," he said.

I knew the first three towns weren't right. "Nope," I said. "Let's go."

"How do you know?" Lee asked. "What are you even looking at?"

"Don't get mad," I told him. "I can just tell. It's a feeling. The way the town *feels*."

Lee rolled his eyes.

When we drove into the fourth town, I sat up straighter. A wooden sign swung above a big storefront with a taffy machine in the window. "NELSON'S CANDY," it said. "Slow down," I told Lee. The old mill town looked captured in time. There was a barbershop, a post office, a five-and-dime called Putnam's, a yoga studio, and an old movie theatre in the town hall that showed classic films on Saturday afternoons. "This might be it," I remember saying.

Lee kept one hand on the wheel and reached into the

backseat with the other. He pulled his arm forward and dropped a pile of papers on my lap. I looked down and saw the real estate listings he must have printed out on our computer. "Wait," I said, "I don't think I'm ready yet." But I couldn't resist taking a quick peek. "Uh oh," I held up a listing. "Two-hundred-year-old historic colonial."

"Call the realtor," Lee said.

"I'm right near there," she told me over the phone. "I can meet you now if you like."

"Uh, hang on a sec." I mouthed to Lee, *right now?*

He smiled and nodded.

"Okay," I told her.

We met Eileen at a nearby gas station and followed her to the house. When she got out of the car, I noticed she wore her gray hair clipped just the way my grandmother had. She had a smudge of lipstick above her right lip.

"I like her," Lee whispered.

"Me too," I whispered back.

I saw the apple trees first, five of them in a little cluster to the right of the driveway. I used to climb the apple tree in our backyard when I was little. Lee liked the old stonewall, separating the yard from the surrounding woods. In the backyard, there was a big hill. "Tuck has always wanted a sledding hill," I said. Eileen took us inside. The house was empty. The owners had moved out two years before when they built a new house. "They're *very* motivated," Eileen said.

We walked from one empty room to the next. Even though the ceilings were cracked and the wallpaper was ancient, the wide pine floorboards and a large fireplace in the living room were wonderful. The house was tall and proud, but it seemed lonely and sad now. I imagined the families that had lived inside these walls for all those years. *Have you been waiting for us?* I asked it silently. Lee walked up and put his arm around me, "I feel like this house has been waiting for us," he said.

Eileen directed us to a nearby school. Just like the house we'd seen, the school was set on a hill and nestled in the woods. I thought we'd just drive by and check it out, but when Lee parked, I got out. We walked through the front doors. In the foyer, a fountain bubbled up from a stone garden. I breathed in the strong smell of cinnamon.

It was a Waldorf school. I'd heard of Waldorf schools but knew nothing about them. We walked down the soft blue hallway, following the sign for the office. I stopped at a glass case to admire the students' work. "First graders knit hats?" I asked. Lee shrugged his shoulders. We walked into the office to request a brochure and the admissions director happened to be at the desk. She also happened to be free and had time for a tour. *Imagine that.*

As she explained the philosophy of Waldorf education, I felt like I had when I learned about holistic medicine. How could these schools exist all over the world for almost a century, and I knew nothing about them? Like holistic medicine's approach of seeing the body as a whole, Waldorf education approaches *the child* as a whole. It teaches children on all levels: mental, physical, emotional, and spiritual.

I thought about when Tucker began kindergarten two years before, how I'd been disillusioned by the school's generic approach to education and said to Lee, "Some days I just want to pick up our family, move north to New Hampshire, and put the kids in some alternative school."

As we drove out of the Waldorf school with our brochures and an appointment to bring the kids back for a visit, I asked Lee if he remembered my saying that. "Of course I do." He smiled. "Hey, you're the one who tells me to be careful, the universe is always listening." I laughed, and leaned back in the seat. *So it is,* I thought.

And just a few short months later, after buckets of tears and heart-breaking goodbyes, we left the only home our children had ever known, the home where Lee and I grew together into adulthood. Maybe it was the way everything lined up, but somehow I knew we were going where we were supposed to be, that as we began a new chapter in our lives in the hills of southern New Hampshire, our healing would occur on an even greater scale. Because in many ways, we still had so much healing to do.

32

Visions

✦

BEFORE WE MADE the final decision to move to New Hampshire, I'd gone back one last time to confirm that we were really on target. We were leaving so much behind, I needed to be certain. I wanted the universe to send us a sign to validate our decision.

It didn't take long. I was passing through the intersection that led to what would soon be our new neighborhood, when a red minivan pulled to a stop. It felt like everything went into slow motion as I drove past. Turning my head, I looked down and caught a glimpse of the license plate: "REIKI."

"No way," I said out loud, shaking my head. There was my sign, and I hadn't even made it to the house.

Reiki was an integral part of our alternative healing practices in Massachusetts. A hands-on Japanese healing technique, Reiki is based on the idea that a vital unseen energy flows through us. The word "Reiki" is a combination of two Japanese words: "rei," meaning "God's wisdom" and "ki," meaning "life force energy." A Reiki practitioner places his or her hands on the body and accesses life force energy to promote healing. It's different for everyone, but for me a Reiki treatment felt like glowing warmth flowing in and around me. Incredibly relaxing, it often led to moments of amazing clarity.

After we moved to New Hampshire I met the driver of this infamous red "Reiki mobile." Libby Barnett, a renowned Reiki master who'd trained thousands throughout her years of practice, lived just down the road from us. At the edge of her driveway stood a big, red mailbox. A picture of a hand was painted on the side.

From the outside, I imagined her yellow Colonial-style home filled with formal furniture and tailored drapes. Yet the inner world was overflowing with enormous crystals, Hindu statues, large comfortable sofas for her weekend classes, and plants gone wild. "It's the Reiki," Libby said, laughing. "The plants love the Reiki." The refrigerator was covered from top to bottom with photos. "That's my David, and there's my Deb." She pointed to photos of graduations, ski trips, and rock climbing adventures. Both kids had her chestnut-colored hair, but hers was short and straight while theirs were long and curly. "They were babies just yesterday, up at the same school where your babies are." She gave me her playful smile. "Now, they're all grown up, about your age." She took my hand in hers. It was so warm. "But it's so good, isn't it? It's all so good."

With her warm and kind way, Libby quickly became a dear friend. Our whole family saw her for appointments. The kids loved their visits. Andie was in awe of the crystals and Tucker loved the mini-trampoline in the living room. Libby's husband, Tom, grew flats of bean sprouts in the kitchen, and after every appointment, Andie left with a plastic bag full. The kids even took an afterschool Reiki class and practiced at home on the dog, the cat, and the guinea pig.

The most incredible, life-changing Reiki session I ever had was in mid-November during the fall after we moved. The air had grown chilly and the days were becoming darker. I had a morning appointment with Libby, but wasn't feeling well and almost canceled. Since I had to get the kids to school anyway, and Lib's house was on the way home, I went.

At the beginning of every appointment, Libby and I always spent several minutes catching up. That day, I began by telling her I wasn't feeling well.

"I don't know what's going on," I said as I sat down across from her in the Reiki room, letting the serene music and slight scent of incense wash over me. "I just feel like shit in an all-over kind of way."

Libby clasped her hands together like an excited child. She loved to play detective in the woes of the body. "So what do you think?" She leaned forward. "Everything okay with the kids and school?"

"Yeah, they love it," I said. "And they're doing really well."

"What about Lee?" Lib asked. "No worries there?"

"Nope," I said.

"Okay, maybe this is about Thanksgiving? Do you have family coming?"

"Just Lee's brother and family," I said. "Which is totally low key."

"Hmmm." She leaned back in her chair with her chin in her hand. Then she popped up. "Let's just get you on the table and see if we can move some stuff around. We'll figure out what's going on."

I climbed on the massage table, and Libby adjusted the pillow under my neck and covered me with a blanket. "Warm enough?" she asked. I nodded. She walked to the end of the table and sat behind my head. Leaning forward, she placed her hands gently on my forehead.

In less than a moment, I knew what was going on. Tears spilled into my hair and onto the pillow "I don't believe it," I said. Libby waited. "Andie's birthday." I wiped the tears from my face in astonishment. "I forgot it's Andie's birthday in two weeks."

Libby kept her hands on my head.

"I can't believe I forgot," I said.

"How old will she be?" Libby asked.

"Seven," I laughed. "She's turning *seven years old.*"

"Wow, seven." Libby placed a hand on my collarbone. Moving around to the left, she put her other hand next to it. I looked up at the framed photo on the wall behind her. A beautiful Indian woman with the deepest, brownest eyes I'd ever seen stared back at me. "In Eastern philosophy, seven is significant," Libby said. "Many believe the body renews itself every seven years." I closed my eyes and pictured Andie's long, graceful frame. "Many also believe the child starts to leave mom's energy field at seven." I opened my eyes and looked up at her. "Your baby's growing up," she said.

Which is all I ever wanted. In the years after Andie had been born, I'd been so conscious of time. My thoughts had been consumed with worry about her future. But in the past few years, I'd seemingly lost track of time. I'd forgotten, but my body had remembered. Every year around the anniversary of Andie's birthday my body relived the trauma and inevitably I had pain or unease in some part of my body.

Libby moved to my middle, just below my belly button. I could feel the heat from her hands. "Take me back through Andie's birth," Libby said. "I know she was born at 25 weeks. But tell me more about it."

I looked out the window where the sun was trying to peer out from behind smoke-colored clouds. Turning back, I noticed for the first time that the lower half of Lib's left eye was the same dark brown as the woman in the photo. "Well," I began, "it was total chaos. For a while we thought we could hold off labor, but Monday morning I had to have an emergency c-section, and Andie was born. I told the nurses I didn't want to see her. They took me anyway."

Libby kept her hands on my abdomen. "Lib," I said. "She was the scariest, ugliest thing I'd ever seen." I couldn't believe I'd said it out loud, but Libby never reacted, she didn't even blink, so I went on. "I didn't want anything to do with her," I said. "I checked out, and Lee had to step up. I just felt like such a failure. I couldn't pump, not even a drop of milk, and I didn't want to know anything about all that medical stuff." I took a big breath and let it out slowly. Libby stayed silent. "Finally, I knew I had to do something. I couldn't stay hidden in that hospital room forever." I closed my eyes, remembering Tasha Tudor on the TV, Lee traveling back and forth to the NICU, and the numerous nurses who watched over Andie. "And then I had this vision," I said, with my eyes still closed. "Two, actually. In one, I saw a funeral and a tiny white casket and all our family dressed in black. In the other vision, I saw this lovely, sassy five-year-old girl, healthy as can be. Obviously I chose the second."

"That's it," Libby spoke so loudly, it scared me. "That's it!" She slapped the side of the table. "You were doing exactly what you were supposed to be doing all along, Kase. You were *holding the vision*."

"Holding the vision?" I opened my eyes.

"Yes." Libby raised both hands in the air like a Southern preacher. "Holding the vision was your job. It was what you were supposed to be doing. That's why you couldn't nurse, and why you didn't care about the medical stuff. You weren't supposed to." Libby put her hands back on my stomach. "All along, you were doing exactly what you were supposed to." She spoke slowly, emphasizing each word. "You were holding the vision of a healthy, strong beautiful girl." She gave me a wide, crinkly-eyed smile. "And look at her today."

I lay in stunned silence. The possibility that everything Libby said was right slowly sank into my system. "That's all I was supposed to do?" I asked. "Hold the vision?"

"Yup." She nodded. "That's all you were supposed to do."

"I did." I put my hands on top of Libby's. "I really did. I saw the vision of that healthy, whole little girl every single day."

And then the strangest thing happened. It was like a giant bubble burst through my middle. I watched as this gush of air flew out of me, over to the window, and outside. "Oh my goodness," I said. "Did you feel that?"

"I did." Lib nodded.

"It's guilt," I said through tears. "It's finally leaving. I didn't know I was still carrying all that stuff around inside me."

"Let it go," Libby said.

"It's gone," I said. "It's gone."

"Phew." Libby wiped her forehead. "That was something."

We both took in several deep breaths and stayed silent.

"I feel different," I finally said.

"I'm sure you do!" Libby laughed.

"I feel free. Like anything's possible."

"You should," Libby said. "You've let so much go."

At the end of the appointment, I gave Libby a big hug of thanks. "So now that I'm not carrying all that junk around, what am I supposed to do with the rest of my life?"

"I don't know," Libby smiled. "Maybe you'll write a book."

"Yeah, I'll get right on that."

We laughed.

"You never know," she said as I walked out the door. "Anything's possible."

✦

That night I had a dream. In the dream, I had just given birth to Andie, but she was bigger and healthier. Even though I was sure I couldn't nurse her, I picked her up and decided to try anyway. When I moved her toward my breast, she latched on immediately. It was so natural. I looked down to see the whitest, creamiest milk on her slightly parted lips. I had the same success when I moved her to the other breast. "Tucker," I called out. "Go get Daddy. I have big news. I nursed Andie."

When I woke up, I knew with certainty that I had *nursed* Andie. Out of curiosity, I looked it up in *Webster's Dictionary*. To nurse: "to take special care of; nourish, foster, develop or cherish." With forgiveness for myself for that horrible time, I finally had the ability to see that, even without one drop of milk, I'd done just that.

33

Trees

✦

THE YEAR TUCKER STARTED third grade he also
started constantly clearing his throat. Not in a subtle
way either. It began like a regular throat clearing and ended
loud, high, and startling. The noise came from deep down
and sounded like something out of a video game or an engine
with a loose fan belt.

On the first day of school, I sat in the auditorium balcony as the first graders were introduced. Each first grader,
including Andie, crossed the stage to receive a rose from an
eighth grader. The room was completely quiet except for the
loud echo of Tucker's throat clearing coming from the student section below. I watched parents shift in their seats, and
kids turn to look at him. My cheeks burned. Looking over
the balcony rail, I studied him, his thick brown hair parted
and combed to the side, his button-down shirt halfway untucked, and his legs swinging back and forth in the khaki
pants he'd worn just for that day. Part of me wanted to go
down, pick him up, and hold him close on my lap. The other
part of me wanted to grab him, shake him, and scream, "Stop
making that noise!" I kept watching him. With his wide eyes,
he followed Andie wherever she moved on the stage.

In first grade Tucker's teacher had sent a note home saying that he was clearing his throat a lot. "It's disturbing the

class," her note said. She suggested we put him on an anti-histamine. Instead, we'd taken him to his pediatrician to rule out acid reflux and throat disorders. The noise soon faded away, but now it was back, and it was worse than ever.

I called Tuck's new pediatrician. After an appointment with her and a referral to an ear, nose, and throat specialist, we all agreed it was a nervous tick. "Very common in boys this age to develop some kind of nervous outlet," his doctor said. "I wouldn't worry, he'll grow out of it."

At home, while the kids played outside, I sat at the kitchen table and called Tucker's teacher, Darcy Drayton. "I am so sorry he's disturbing the class. This is so upsetting."

"Kasey," she said, "I think you're more upset about this than you need to be."

Darcy explained how she'd pulled Tuck aside and asked his permission to talk to the class about the noise. The children had an open discussion about the different things they do when they feel nervous. "I think it was a wonderful learning experience for the entire class, and Tucker feels really supported by his classmates."

"Thank you," was all I could mutter or I would have started crying in relief. "Tucker's very well adjusted on the outside." She paused. I could hear her choosing her words carefully. "But inside there seems to be some underlying sorrow. Some apprehension."

Out the window I could see Tucker pushing Andie on the swing. "I think he carries some of the trauma of Andie's birth inside him," I said.

"What about painting therapy?" Darcy's voice sounded

hopeful. "It would be a wonderful way to help him bring those stuck emotions to the surface."

So for eight weeks Tucker met once a week with a beautiful, soft-spoken Danish woman named Karine (pronounced kuh-ree-nuh). "The goal of the painting," Karine told me over coffee one morning, "is to bring those veiled emotions within Tucker to light. Move him through color, so he can leave those dark hues behind and begin to be in the bright, fire colors, you know?"

I nodded. That sounded good to me.

At the end of the eight weeks, Tucker pulled a folded invitation out of his backpack and handed it to me.

"What's this?" I asked.

He picked up his skateboard, ready to head outside. "I'm all done with my paintings." He smiled. "We're going to have a party and you and Daddy can see them."

"That's awesome, bud." I tacked the invitation to the bulletin board. "Daddy and I would love to come." As he bounced out the door with his skateboard, I realized that I hadn't heard that throat clearing noise in at least a week.

✦

We met Karine at school in her studio behind the auditorium. Lee and I waited in the dim hallway with Darcy while Karine and Tucker finished setting up. "Almost ready," Karine called. When the door opened, Tucker was standing just inside, his apple-red cheeks and proud smile reminded me of the first time he held Andie in the hospital. As we walked in, he took our hands in his. The table was covered in a light pink cloth. On it was a lit candle, homemade rolls and jam, juice, and coffee cake. "Oh, Karine, this is beautiful," I said.

"Well, Tucker is a special boy, and he's done such a wonderful job, we just had to celebrate, you know?"

"I know," I said.

The three of us sat down while Tuck took his place next to an easel. Karine sat in a chair at his side. "Tucker has decided he wants to hold up his paintings, while I read the story he wrote, okay?"

As Tucker pulled the first painting off the easel, Lee reached over and took my hand.

The story began with a bear in a cave, at night, deep in the forest. The accompanying watercolors were done in shadowy blues, purples, and blacks. As the story progressed, Tucker's color choices moved from cool, deep colors to warm, fiery reds, yellows, and oranges.

The paintings chronicled the bear's awakening from his long winter hibernation. He came out of the cave to investigate this new world and spent a long day exploring. After a while, he was tired and eager to go back to his cave. Upon returning, however, he found he could not go back because the forest was on fire. In Tucker's words, "The fire happened because things like that happen in real life." Lee squeezed my hand tighter. "The bear had to be very brave and search for a new home," Karine read. "The bear climbed the tallest green hill. He looked over the great open world. He felt hopeful. He was tired but happy. There was a brother and a sister tree that were both full of lush green leaves. In between, the bear found a mossy bed that fit him perfectly. He lay down under the two trees and fell fast asleep. He dreamt good dreams. He was safe."

As the story ended, I could no longer hold back my tears, and I reached for a napkin on the table. Tucker set his paintings down, walked over, and wrapped his arms around my neck. Lee put his arms around both of us. We stayed that way for several moments.

"I made my Danish rolls," Karine finally said.

We all laughed.

After Mrs. Drayton and Tucker headed back to the classroom, we stayed and spoke to Karine for a few minutes more. She pushed her long blond hair behind her shoulders. "He's a lovely little boy, you know?"

"Well, he really loves you," I said.

"It was so cute," she said. "When we were setting up the table, he said, 'You did all this for me?' When I told him, 'Yes, all for you,' he said, 'Wow, a teacher gave me a Hershey kiss once, but that was all.'"

Lee and I smiled at each other.

"He obviously trusted you," I said. "You really got him to open up."

Karine fingered the beads around her neck. "I want to tell you one more thing before you go," she said. "At the end of the story, with the two trees, the brother and sister trees, you remember?"

We both nodded.

"Well, Tucker painted the first tree, big and tall with lots of leaves. 'That's the brother tree,' he told me. He painted the second tree, this one smaller and leafless. 'That's the sister tree,' he'd said. 'She doesn't have any leaves.'" Karine stopped for a moment and dabbed at her eyes. "So I look at him and say, 'Oh, but Tucker, don't you see? The sister tree does have all her leaves.' He looked at me with those big eyes, you know? And then he said, 'Oh yeah, you're right. She does have all her leaves.' And he went on to finish his painting, covering the sister tree with those emerald green leaves."

I looked at the painting resting on the wooden easel and just for a moment could have sworn I saw those leaves rustle in the breeze.

✦

Just days after sharing his paintings, Tucker was sitting with Andie in the overstuffed chair by the kitchen window. It was late afternoon, but I was only just starting to wash the griddle from the morning pancakes. The kids leaned into each other as they read their books. Tucker was reading *The Cricket in Times Square* and Andie was in her *Henry and Mudge* phase. Classical music played from the radio on the counter. Without warning, Tucker looked up from his book and turned to Andie. "Did you know you almost died?" he asked. I froze and then carefully set down the griddle and shut off the water so I could hear.

Andie looked up. "Yeah, I know," she said. "That was when I was a baby."

Tucker shoved her over to claim a little more chair space, "Yeah," he said, "When you were a baby." And with that they both went back to reading their books.

34

Steps

✦

IT WAS LATE AUTUMN, and Lee and I were sitting in little student chairs across from Andie's teacher, Susan Schickel. Sunlight poured through the tall windows of her first grade classroom, and a pink geranium climbed the side of the windowsill. Vibrant student paintings hung on the walls, and a wooden tree house in the corner waited for visiting fairies and gnomes. Susan's clothes were tidy and pressed. I wondered what her family was doing that Saturday while she stayed at school, hosting parent conferences.

"Andie's doing really well," Susan said. Whenever she spoke about Andie, her voice was soft and kind. "And she's a delight to have in class." She showed us examples of her schoolwork from a folder with Andie's name printed across the top. Then she placed the folder on the floor next to her chair and folded her hands in her lap. "So," she said. "Something has come up recently in movement class." She paused.

Lee and I sat up straighter in our chairs.

"We're not overly concerned, but Mrs. Davis, her movement teacher, noticed that Andie is the only one in first grade who isn't skipping." She tucked her hair behind her ear. "It's something we'll continue to work on at school, and we thought you might want to do the same at home."

I heard Karen McCarthy's voice echo in my ears: *As Andie moves forward in school, little things will creep up. They'll be inconsistent with how well she's doing. But just be aware that they are somehow connected to her birth.* When she'd spoken this warning, it meant little to me. Now, I understood. I didn't know why Andie wasn't skipping, but I knew this was a *something* that had come up. As soon as we got home, I called Karen and made an appointment for Andie to see her.

"Long time no see, strangers," Karen called as we climbed out of the warm car into the chilly autumn air. She waited on the porch, dressed in dark corduroys, a white turtleneck, and red wool vest. I took Andie's hand as we walked across the yard. "It's freezing," I said. "Come in, come in." Karen opened the door and pulled Andie in for a hug. "You got big," she said.

"I'm on a soccer team." Andie kicked off her sneakers. "Do you have all the same toys?"

"Sure do," Karen said, "They're down there waiting for you." We watched Andie run down the stairs.

"I am *loving* that this school has such an awareness and focus on body movements," Karen said as we followed Andie. "It's great to be able to discover this now because developmental milestones can build on each other." We stood at the bottom of the stairs, watching Andie roll around on a big, blue exercise ball. "If they hadn't caught this now, it probably would have come up later, in fourth or fifth grade. But by then it would be a different issue, maybe trouble understanding math equations or something."

I pulled out my notebook as Karen continued. "I'm

certain Andie missed some developmental reflex, either in utero or during infancy," she said. "And that's why she's not skipping." As Karen continued, I sat down and began writing. "These reflexes emerge in utero and are present at birth. Reflexes influence motor development and play a certain role in building movement patterns." I looked up from my notebook. "So if a baby isn't in utero for long, if they're born at 25 weeks," I nodded toward Andie, "some of these reflexes aren't matured?"

"Absolutely," Karen sat down on the step next to me. "Think about how long Andie had a pacifier in the hospital. She had to *learn* the sucking reflex that full-term babies already know." I nodded, starting to understand.

"Andie," Karen called to her. "Two more minutes, and then it's time to get started."

"Ohhh," Andie said. "But we just got here." She somersaulted off the ball.

"When these sequential reflexes are missed," Karen said. "Anything can occur, including poor muscle tone, hyperactivity, learning disabilities, even bed-wetting." Karen paused while I scribbled in my notebook.

"I had a 12-year-old girl referred to me," she said, "who still wet her bed almost every night."

I winced.

"Her parents tried everything, and I mean *everything*." Karen blew her bangs out of her eyes. "I helped her explore possible skipped reflexes. After two sessions, she stopped wetting her bed and hasn't done so since."

"That's incredible," I said.

Karen nodded. "It's really powerful work. Simple, but powerful. You'll see." She walked over to Andie and put her foot under the ball to keep it from spinning. "Okay, my dear, two minutes are up."

Andie rolled her eyes in protest.

Karen grinned at her and put her hands on her hips. "One more roll if you promise we'll get right to work after that."

Andie ran over to hand me her glasses. "This is going to be my biggest one yet," she said.

Once the ball was tucked away in a corner, Karen walked to the end of the room. "Okay, Andie," she said. "Skip to me." Andie looked across the room. She lifted her right leg up and forward and set it down. Then she lifted her left leg up, bent it at the knee and stepped forward with a little hop. Her tongue poked out the side of her mouth as she concentrated. Her movements resembled skipping, but they were awkward and forced. Her class was skipping in a circle every morning at school, and Andie was slowly catching on, but without fluidity or rhythm. As she turned back to go across the room again Karen said quietly, "Through sheer will and determination she's figured out a way to skip, but it's not integrated in any way within her body."

Once Andie was on the massage table, Karen started moving her legs in and out and side to side. I grabbed my notebook off the chair as Karen explained the reflex she believed Andie had missed. "You know how you step on a rock with one foot?" Karen took a step forward and then stopped as if she'd just stepped on something sharp. "What do you do?" she asked.

I stared at her, waiting for the answer. When one didn't come I pretended to step on a rock and said, "You shift your weight, or hop onto the other foot, or skip?"

"Precisely," Karen said. "That reflex is called leg cross flexion-extension reflex. It emerges six months in utero and one to two months after birth." She turned to Andie, put her hands on Andie's legs, and starting tickling. Andie squirmed and shrieked. "Okay, you. Ready to do a little work?" Karen asked.

For the next 15 minutes, I watched Karen move Andie's skinny legs around. When she pushed Andie's leg one way, Andie concentrated hard and pushed back with all her might. They made a game of who could groan louder. Finally Karen said, "Okay, hop off the table, and let me see you skip across the room."

Andie jumped off the table. Then she gracefully skipped from one end of the room to the other as if she'd been doing it all her life. She turned around with a big smile on her face and skipped back to me. Back in her two-year-old days, she'd say "clap for me mommy!" after any new achievement. I wanted to clap but didn't want to embarrass her. Instead I gave her a big hug and whispered in her ear, "I'm happy for you, Andie Lou."

She pushed out of the hug. "Can I go back to the ball now?" she asked.

"If you skip over to it," Karen said from the doorway.

We watched her skip, beautifully, over to the ball.

I turned to Karen. "Do you know how many times I've left this office stunned and amazed?" I asked. "What did you just do?"

She sat down on the arm of the chair across from me. "Well, essentially the exercises I took Andie through gave her brain and central nervous system a second chance to learn what it missed the first time."

We looked over at Andie, rolling on the ball. "Karen, you are amazing," I said.

"No." She nodded to Andie. "She's amazing."

Andie looked up and gave us a big smile.

"You're amazing, Andie Lou," I called over.

"I know," she said.

And we all laughed.

35

Margaritas

✦

I WAS RAISED CATHOLIC. My Episcopalian mom stayed home or went to her church on Sunday mornings while my brother, sister, and I squished in the backseat of the wood-paneled station wagon and complained about having to go to 10:30 mass. At 10:40, dad drove us into the parking lot, and that's when his Sunday morning prayers would begin. "Jesus Christ," he'd call out, "there are no parking spots." Gripping the wheel tighter, he'd look up. "Please God, I'm a hard-working guy who doesn't ask for much. Just find me a goddamn parking space." We'd end up at the farthest end of the lot near the cemetery. After suffering through Dad's pleas to walk faster, we'd slip into the congregation hall to the stares and glares of the already seated churchgoers.

Long before we got married in a traditional church ceremony, Lee declared our church to be "the church of the two planks," aka: skis. He wanted our wedding vows to read, "To love, honor, and ski," but I'd drawn the line there. Our house in Massachusetts was next door to the Catholic church, and on Sundays (when we weren't skiing), we'd sit on the front porch in our pajamas, eating pancakes and waving to friends as they walked to morning mass. At six months old, we dressed Tucker in navy linen shorts, a white button-down shirt, and a clip-on bow tie, and took him to the church where I'd been baptized. I'd forgotten his shoes, so he was baptized in little white tube socks.

When Andie was in the NICU, some families had their fragile babies baptized right there in their plastic isolettes, amid beeping alarms and glaring fluorescent lights. We never did that, and once Andie came home, church became a terrifying haven of germs, a crowd of living, breathing humans who threatened her very existence. As she got older and healthier, we attended the Congregational church once a year on Christmas Eve so the kids could dress up as animals in the nativity pageant.

The closest church in New Hampshire was a good ten-minute drive from our new house, and since we'd never had much church in our past, I felt quite certain we wouldn't have much church in our future. Until we met our new neighbors, the Owens.

Their daughter, Helen, was in Andie's class and their son, Burton, was just a year older than Tucker. Originally from Tennessee, Eleanor was a one-woman welcome wagon. The first time we met, she greeted me with a hug. "We're so glad y'all are here." She had a little ski jump nose and pretty brown eyes that got big from excitement when she talked. "How about we have a cookout for y'all Saturday?" That cookout with the Owens would be the first of many.

We drove over with our kids and a case of beer. Their house was old, like ours. A white picket fence and a well-tended garden led the way to the back door, and their mudroom was filled with gardening shoes, riding boots, soccer cleats, and baseball gloves.

Eleanor opened the door wearing a sundress and a white

cardigan buttoned just at the top. "Y'all made it." She gave
me a big hug. "Come in, come in," she said. "Everyone is out
in the yard."

Andie and Tucker ran outside to play while Lee deposit-
ed the beer into a metal tub already filled with lemonade and
seltzer. I followed Eleanor into the kitchen. A tall red-haired
man wearing paint-splattered shorts came through the porch
door, carrying a platter of hamburgers and hot dogs. "Chris
Owen," he said, shifting the platter to his left hand and ex-
tending his right so we could shake.

"Thanks for having us," I said. "Your house is beautiful."

Behind me, Lee was still clanking bottles in the tub.

"What brought you to the area?" Chris asked.

I nodded toward the clanking sound. "My husband's job."

Chris smiled. There was a pause.

"Where do you work?" I asked.

He set the platter down on the table. "The Congregational
church."

"*Oh.*" I might have taken a step back. "What do you do
there?"

"I'm the minister," he said.

"The minister." The bottles were still clanking in the
background, and suddenly they sounded very loud. "Leave
it to us to show up at the minister's house with an overabun-
dance of beer."

Chris and Eleanor laughed. "Please," she drawled. "I'm
a Southern woman who drinks and cusses with the best of
'em." She took my arm and led me over to Lee. "Let's have
ourselves a beer."

Soon Eleanor and I were talking on the phone every

morning. We walked together, swapped books, and drove each other's kids back and forth to school. One night while sitting in bed and recalling the days events, most of them involving Eleanor, Lee said, "Look's like you've got yourself a girlfriend."

"I know it," I said. "And here I thought I'd be sitting all alone on top of this hill."

"I'm proud of you." He leaned over and kissed me on the cheek.

"*For making a friend?*" I said.

"For being open to the possibility." He patted my hand.

◆

Tucker and Burton had become fast friends, and that fall, Lee coached their soccer team. We called them the "dynamic duo" on the field. Andie and Helen, an inseparable pair, cheered the boys on when they weren't playing in their own soccer games. At the end of the season the Owens treated us to a Mexican dinner as a celebration and thank you to Coach Lee.

We sat in Amigos, the local Mexican restaurant, at a table for eight surrounded by brightly woven rugs, piñatas, and strands of red chili pepper lights. Baskets of chips and salsa arrived and we rearranged seats so the boys could see the Red Sox on the bar TV.

"To new friends and soccer," Lee said. The kids clinked their glasses of root beer. We did the same with our margaritas.

"So," I set my drink down on the table and turned to Chris. "You're a minister."

"I *am* a minister," Chris said, putting his hand on his chest and raising his eyebrows.

"Then this is a school night for you," Lee said.

Chris laughed. "Yup, Saturday night is my school night."

"So what do you *do* as a minister?" I asked.

"Kasey." Lee shook his head.

"What?" I asked. "I just want to know."

To Lee's embarrassment, I conducted an informal interview throughout the meal, satiating my curiosity about Chris's choice of profession. "You're a busy man," I said after listening to him explain some of his duties, which include his Sunday service, visits to sick parishioners, performing marriages and funerals, attending budget meetings, and offering counseling. "And occasionally fixin' a leaky pipe," Eleanor added.

By the end of the evening, I knew how and why he'd become a minister and all about his routine of preparing his weekly sermon at the local coffee shop. "We should come and listen to you some Sunday," I said as he signaled for the check.

Lee and Eleanor were involved in their own conversation. "Lee," I elbowed him. "Do you want to check out Chris's church?"

"Uh, yeah . . . sure," he said, rubbing his forehead.

Later, after putting our exhausted kids to bed, Lee said, "What did you do that for?"

I climbed under the covers with him. "Do what?"

"Say we'd go to church."

"I didn't say we'd *go to church.*" I fluffed up my pillow like I did every night, which drove Lee crazy. "I said *maybe* we'd check it out sometime."

"Well, now we'll have to go."

"Yeah, we will," I said.

"Tomorrow," Lee said.

"*Tomorrow?*" I sat up in bed. "I'm not going to church tomorrow."

"Kasey, you basically interrogated the guy all night. It would be rude if we didn't go tomorrow."

"It won't be rude."

"We're going."

"Fine." I rolled over and closed my eyes. "We'll get it over with."

We had trouble finding the church. By the time we arrived, we were late. Chris was standing at the altar, dressed in a long black robe. He smiled when we walked in. Helen turned to see who he was smiling at, and her freckled face lit up when she saw us. She tapped Eleanor, who motioned for us to sit with them *in the front row.* As we walked down the aisle, people offered smiles.

"Welcome friends and guests. It is good to gather together," Chris began.

After we sat down, I looked around at the old white church. Sunlight poured through the huge windows. Music played. Voices sang. Lee took my hand.

"And now," Chris said. "If all the children would come forward." Andie and Tucker followed Helen and Burton into the aisle with the other kids. They gathered at Chris's feet. I can't remember what he talked about, but I remember he spoke softly and looked at each child, laughing when one said something funny.

After the children left for Sunday school, Chris began

his sermon. *That* I remember. He spoke about peace and love and how we must first find these things in ourselves before we can find them elsewhere in the world. It echoed a conversation I'd had with Libby Barnett earlier that week during a Reiki session.

That morning my notion of church was turned on its head and for the rest of the fall we went to church regularly. When snow started flying, we headed to the mountains, but as soon as ski season was over, we were back at church in the spring. On our way out the doors one Sunday in early April, I turned to Lee. "I want Chris to baptize Andie."

Lee put his arm around me. "I do, too," he said.

♦

We chose a late Sunday in May. Chris asked us to meet him before the christening so we could go over details and expectations. On a spring morning when the dogwoods were in bloom, we found ourselves sitting in the living room of our dear friend and minister, Chris Owen. I knew the room well. I'd helped Eleanor choose the fabric for the chairs. I knew the stories behind most of the antique furniture. "This was Mamma's," she'd say. "And this was Aunt Jane's, and this was Daddy's favorite chair."

That morning Eleanor stayed in the kitchen, brewing coffee while Chris asked us why we wanted to have Andie baptized. I answered for both of us, explaining that in the past we'd done things because it was what we were supposed to do. We'd been right on schedule with the whole college, job, marriage, and baby thing. Tucker had been baptized at six months in the same Catholic Church I'd gone to as a child because that's what we were *supposed* to do. But this time, I told Chris, we were *choosing* to have Andie baptized because she was healthy and alive, and it felt like the right time. "She's seven," I said. "It's time to celebrate and acknowledge her."

"Seven," Chris said.

We sat in silence for a few moments. "I know about Andie's birth," he finally said. "But if you will, take me back through that time."

I spoke about my guilt and fear and Lee's incredible strength.

Chris turned to Lee, who was sitting next to me on the camelback sofa. "I'm wondering, Lee," Chris rubbed his chin, "Where you found the strength to get through that difficult time."

Lee leaned forward, rested his elbows on his knees, and told the story of our friends, Holly and Fletch. Their first child, Ford, was born just months after Tucker. Because of his severe disabilities, he would live a mere five weeks. During that time, Fletcher continued to make his residency rounds, delivering babies, and visiting his son in the NICU.

"During one visit," Lee said. "Fletcher placed his forehead on Ford's and asked, 'Why are you here? What are you here to teach me?'" Lee cleared his throat. "Fletch told me that he heard it clearly, an immediate response, transmitted directly back. 'Unconditional love,' his son told him. 'I'm here to teach you unconditional love.'" Lee wiped his eyes and sat up straighter. "And that's where I found my strength."

"Unconditional love," Chris repeated, barely aloud.

"Yeah," Lee said. "Unconditional love."

On that Sunday in May when Chris baptized Andie, the sun shone the entire day. Andie wore a beautiful white dress, a white bow in her hair, and sparkly silver shoes. Our entire family showed up. Chris called all the children forward to bless the holy water before it anointed Andie's head. After the service we took pictures outside the church and then went back to our house for a celebration. We abandoned the idea of a traditional brunch with tea sandwiches and fruit salad and, because it was *our* choice, opted instead to begin a new baptismal tradition of burgers, beers, and a backyard bouncy house.

Hallelujah!

36

Talents

✦

IT WAS A QUIET SATURDAY AFTERNOON in September. Lee was in the garage working on his car, the kids were playing upstairs, and I was wrapped in a quilt, reading a book on the living room couch. The smell from the pot of soup simmering on the stove drifted toward me, and I suddenly felt hungry. Looking up from my book, I realized it had gotten very quiet. I was about to go check on the kids when I heard pounding footsteps on the stairs. Tucker always took every stair as if making an important point. When he reached the bottom step, he made his final two-footed jump and then ran into the living room, wearing his navy pajama bottoms and a long-sleeved skateboarding shirt. He was out of breath, wild eyed, and panting. My stomach clenched. *Something happened to Andie*, I thought, but then his face broke into a big grin, and I let out the breath I was holding and sank back into the couch.

"Mom." Tucker took a big breath. "You're not going to believe this."

I waited.

"We discovered Andie's talent!" He took another breath and raised his hands in the air. "She has a talent."

"That's wonderful, honey." I stifled a laugh.

More pounding footsteps from the stairway. It sounded

like Andie was jumping down with both feet together on every step. The pounding stopped when she reached the bottom. Tucker peeked around the corner of the living room door.

"Ready, Andie?" he asked. He looked back into the room, his eyes wide as he rocked back and forth on his toes. "Are *you* ready, Mom?"

I tried to match his serious tone. "I'm ready, Tuck."

"Okay." He stood up tall and swept the room with one arm in a grand gesture. "Presenting, Andie!" He walked out of the room. When he returned, Andie was in front of him, jumping forward with each step. Tucker held his hands on both of her shoulders, guiding her toward me. From her shoulders to her ankles, her long, skinny body was covered in tightly buckled belts. With her arms bound behind her back, she gave me an enormous smile. Tucker, the little ringmaster, announced to his crowd of one, "Fourteen belts!" He turned Andie around in a circle. Underneath the belts, she was wearing her horsey pajamas. *"She is wrapped in 14 belts!"*

He paused for dramatic effect. I widened my eyes and mouthed an amazed "Wow."

"Okay," he continued. "Here she goes folks." He wiped his mouth with the back of his hand. "Ready, Andie. 1, 2, 3 . . . go!"

And there, before my eyes, in a few brief moments, my little Houdini managed to wriggle her way out of the entanglement of belts. Her bony shoulders twisted and wriggled, and her arms moved to the front of her body. The belts began sliding down over her thin hips. As the last one fell to the floor, they raised their arms in the air together and shouted, "Ta-da!" in unison.

My first inclination was to ask where they'd found all those belts and what the upstairs bedrooms looked like. Instead, I hollered "Hooray! Bravo! Bravisimo!" I whistled and clapped.

Both kids bowed.

Tucker, Andie's stage manager and promoter, patted her on the back. "Great job, Andie. That's an awesome talent." Satisfied with his protégé, he scampered back upstairs. What he was onto next I didn't dare guess.

Andie stepped over the belts and ran to me. She climbed onto the couch and curled her back up against my front. I hugged her body and breathed in the smell of her hair. Her heart beat fast against my arm. "Mom?" she said, pulling her knees toward her chest.

"Yeah?"

She seemed to hesitate.

"What is it, honey?" I asked.

She turned and looked up at me with her big, earnest eyes. "Do you . . ." she started, then began again as if she wanted to get the words just right. "Do you really think that I have a talent?"

I looked down at her, her blond hair fanned out behind her and her pink, pouty lips parted slightly under that delicate nose and high round cheekbones. I thought of her miniscule, barely there body at birth. I thought of the surgeries, the stitches, and the statistics. I thought of the impossibility that she'd turn out to be this unbelievably amazing child. I replayed the image of her wriggling out of those belts and realized she'd gotten herself out of much tighter situations than that.

"Yeah," I said softly, touching her chin. "I think that you have a talent."

She smiled.

"I think you have many, many talents."

Pushing up on her elbows, she kissed me on the lips. Then she curled further into my side, and I pulled her even closer. *My girl. My remarkably talented girl.*

37

Possibility

◆

THAT FALL Andie started second grade, the grade I'd taught before having children of my own. Her eighth birthday was fast approaching. For months I'd been promising a research assistant at Children's Hospital that I'd bring her back to Boston. They wanted to follow up on the brain study she was enrolled in just after her birth. The appointment would involve a few hours of cognitive tests. They would use the results to study the long-term effects on children who experienced a brain bleed while in the NICU. I kept meaning to schedule it, but Andie's school days were long, and then she had riding lessons and soccer practice, and everything seemed to take precedence over a neurological exam.

Finally, after the research assistant left yet another message, I called back and scheduled an appointment for the second week in November, the week before her birthday. It seemed an auspicious time, and it would be my chance to take her to the Isabella Stewart Gardner Museum, as I'd always wanted to do. When I told Andie our plans for the day, she clapped her hands and gave me a big hug. "Just us?" she asked.

"Yup. It'll be a girl's day out." I tucked her hair behind her ear. "An early birthday celebration."

During her appointment at Children's, Andie played "games" with three different research doctors. They'd been following her progress for years, but as the tests progressed and the questions became harder, they raised their eyebrows in surprise. She answered each one successfully.

Toward the end of the appointment the study's lead neurologist arrived, dressed just as he had been when we'd first met him in the NICU, black cowboy boots poking out from under black jeans, his curly brown hair hanging to the shoulders of his white lab coat. "How are you doing, Andie?" His foreign accent was charming. He'd once told me where he was from, but I'd forgotten. He examined Andie and then leaned against the counter, flipping through pages of test results while the research assistant gave her a small bag of gifts. I stood near the door, watching Andie and the assistant looking through a sheet of stickers at the little round table. The neurologist walked over and stood by my side. "She's truly amazing."

I nodded.

"So many other babies in the study . . ." He ran his hand through his hair. "The struggles they're facing . . ." his voice trailed off. "One of the problems is that there's a lack of services for these kids because they don't fall under any category of disability, there's no standard label for them." I watched Andie explain the rules of a mini-board game to the assistant. "I just can't emphasize how well Andie has done," he said. For several moments we stood watching her in silence.

I surprised myself when I broke the silence. "I have my own theories about Andie's success," I said.

He turned to me, his brown eyes waiting. I hesitated. Was

I really going to lecture a top Boston neurologist? I watched Andie take a star sticker and put it on her new pad of paper, and then I began to tell him about the alternative therapies we'd used to complement mainstream care. My voice grew stronger and more confident as I spoke. I told him about energy work, the cranial-sacral therapy, Reiki, and the power of intention.

When I finished I let out a big breath. He had his arms crossed over his chest. He seemed to be studying the tips of his black cowboy boots. I had no idea what he would say, until he nodded. "There's so much we don't know," he said. In a quieter voice he added, "I think you're right. We have to start exploring alternative paths if we want these babies to turn out like her." He nodded to Andie, who was spinning a small top around the table, putting her hand up every time it threatened to spin off the side.

"You know," I told him. "Probably the best thing we did was the dark blanket thing."

He frowned. "The dark blanket thing?"

"It was really just a stroke of luck," I began. And then I went on to explain how early on a nurse had suggested we bring a blanket in from home so we could cover Andie's isolette and block out the light and noise from the NICU. Lee's mom happened to grab the heavy, navy blue blanket off the back of our living room couch. That blanket covered Andie's isolette throughout her time in the NICU. Late one night, nearly a year after Andie arrived home, I couldn't sleep so I sprawled out on the living room couch to watch television. Curling up under that same navy blanket, I flipped through several channels, settling on a PBS show on brain development that I figured would put me right to sleep.

Instead, I was jolted awake. A doctor from the very hospital where Andie was born was talking about a research study she conducted with premature infants. In a thick German accent she explained her hypothesis that the fragile, still-developing brains of these preemies needed a quiet, womb-like environment in order to heal and grow. I sat up and looked at the blanket that had created that quiet, dark place for Andie. So many other babies had lain under white receiving blankets, or nothing at all.

Later, I learned the program was called *The Secret Life of the Brain*. The doctor, who was working to change NICU environments, was named Dr. Heidelise Als. From then on, whenever I received a phone call from a friend of a friend who had just delivered a premature baby and desperately wanted to know what they could do for them, I'd think of Dr. Als and say, "Get them a thick, dark blanket."

"Mom, look," Andie held up a Winnie the Pooh notebook covered in stickers.

"Wow!" I told her.

The neurologist was rubbing his chin. "I think most of the NICUs are starting to dim the lights and keep things quieter."

I nodded. "I hope so," I told him. I watched Andie packing up her new gifts and thought of all those undeveloped babies, born before they were ready. Like little plant seedlings, they belonged in dark, warm soil where they could absorb nourishment and rest until they were ready to seek the light and emerge above the surface.

"I'm all done." Andie walked over, holding her gift bag at her side. The neurologist squatted down until he was at Andie's eye level. He put both his hands on her shoulders. "I want to thank you for coming all the way down here today, Andie," he said. "I hope someday all of the babies born so small and fragile will grow up to be as big and strong as you."

Andie held his gaze. "You're welcome," she said. Then she leaned in closer like she had a secret to share. The doctor leaned forward to meet her. "By the way," she said, "your games are really boring."

That sweet doctor threw back his head and laughed and laughed. "You're right," he said at last. "They're not much fun at all."

After we said goodbye, we walked out the door, hand in hand, down the hospital corridor until we got to the elevators. When I turned around, I saw our cowboy neurologist was still standing in the doorway, watching us.

✦

Andie and I sat on the stone steps next to the courtyard at the Isabella Stewart Gardner Museum. It was the exact spot where I'd sat seven years before. "This stone is warm," Andie said, pressing her palm into the granite.

I pointed up to the glass ceiling. "The sun," I said. I watched Andie look around in amazed silence, absorbing the incredible beauty before her eyes. Exotic emerald and jade plants climbed up the filigreed cornices, garden paths wound around ivory-colored statues, and angelic faces emerged out of the old stone walls.

I turned when I heard the sound of heels clicking on the floor behind us. An older woman in low black pumps, a wool plaid skirt, and pearls walked up behind us. Her badge said, "VOLUNTEER."

"Good afternoon, ladies." She had a deep Julia Child–type voice that made me smile. She cleared her throat. "I couldn't help but notice how absorbed you and your charming daughter are in our marvelous courtyard." She turned to gaze at the vast greenery. When she turned back, she seemed to have forgotten what she was going to say. "Ah, yes," she fingered her pearls. "I was wondering if your lovely daughter would like the sketching paper and clipboard we volunteers have put together for our young visitors."

Andie nodded shyly.

"That would be nice," I said.

"Very good." The woman clapped her hands together. I watched her walk over to a desk where another older woman passed her a clipboard. Bending down, she offered the clipboard to Andie.

"Thank you," Andie said quietly.

"My pleasure," she said in her robust voice.

I watched her walk back to her station at the volunteer desk. Andie picked up the pencil and started sketching one of the statues. When her blond hair fell across her face, I drew it back and tucked it behind her ear.

"It's so beautiful here," Andie said.

"So beautiful." I nodded. But I wasn't looking at the

courtyard; I was looking at her delicate, perfectly formed features.

Eventually we pulled ourselves away from the courtyard and started toward the galleries. Passing the volunteer desk, the two older women asked to see Andie's drawing. "Why, she's an artist," said the one who'd brought over the clipboard.

I pulled Andie into my side for a little hug. "She's a talented girl," I said.

"Enjoy your tour," the woman told us. "It's all as Isabella left it."

The other woman nodded. "That was part of the agreement. She bequeathed her home as a museum as long as everything remained just as she had it."

"Amazing," I said.

The women looked pleased.

Andie and I began walking up the stone steps to the second floor. A red tapestry the size of a huge living room rug hung on the wall. Andie stopped and looked closer. "Wow," her eyes widened. "It must be really old."

At the top of the stairs we entered the first room. On my first visit, I'd never made it to the galleries, and now I found the gold-framed oil paintings, dark wooden furniture, and deep red walls intimidating, a little scary. But Andie was enchanted. She walked right into the room. I followed her as she led the way from room to room. When she stopped to study each priceless work of art, I studied her.

The rooms wound around until finally we were in the last room at the top of the stairs. Andie crossed the floor to an enormous painting of Isabella Stewart Gardner hanging in the corner. "Is that her?" She glanced back at me.

I stepped closer to read the plaque, but the female security guard standing next to the door answered first. "That's her alright."

Andie traced her finger along the plaque. "John Singer Sargent," she read. "Was he the painter?"

"Yes, he was the painter," I answered. I followed Andie as she moved along the wall, studying each painting. When we got to two large wooden frames, she stopped. "They're empty," she said, taking my hand.

"They are." I remembered the newspaper headlines from all those years ago when the paintings had been stolen. I looked over at the security guard. "Are these the paintings that were stolen?" I asked.

"Two of them," she said.

"Why are the frames still hanging, empty like this?" I asked.

"Gotta leave everything just like it was when Mrs. Gardner passed. Paintings or no paintings, that's where she hung 'em, that's where they gotta stay."

"Huh," I turned back to join Andie, who was still looking into the empty space inside the dark frames.

She looked up at me with a worried crease across her brow and asked, "Will they ever put those paintings back?"

"I don't know, sweetie," I said.

Looking up at the framed, blank wall, I thought about all that had been stolen from our family: the joy of a full pregnancy, those blissful days right after a baby arrives when she's just waking up to the world, the sweet closeness of nursing. As a newborn, Andie never experienced the difference between night and day, she never felt the light breeze blowing on her baby face, a dog's thick coat beneath her baby hand, or the sound of her first autumn leaves rustling in the wind. I stared into that empty space. She'd also been robbed of a mother who was delighted, rather than terrified, every time she looked into her baby's eyes.

I glanced down at Andie. Who would have thought we could make it through such a vicious journey? From premature baby to vibrant eight-year-old. We knew so much more now than ever before; we knew Andie had an enduring core, a survivalist's disposition. We knew that her brother would clear any obstacle blocking her path and that her Dad would remain devoted to her just as he had been from the very beginning. And we knew, too, that in her darkest hour, her mother could learn to emerge from pain and find out what strength was. Most of all, we knew that through a series of what felt like miracles, Andie had gotten a second chance at living in this wild, wonderful world where nothing is impossible.

"You know what, Andie Lou?" I ran a finger down her nose. "They just might get those paintings back." She looked up at me with wide hopeful eyes. "You never can tell," I told her. "Anything . . . anything is possible."

✦

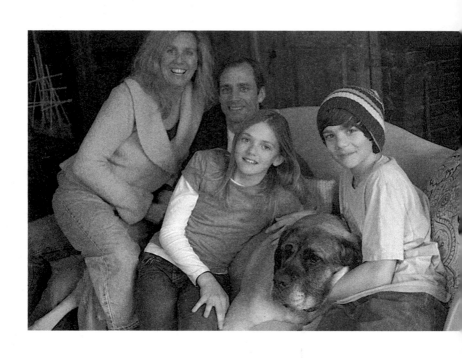

Epilogue

+

C. S. LEWIS ONCE WROTE that girls grow faster than books. As this book nears publication, Andie is 11 years old. I guess Mr. Lewis was right!

At her 11-year-old pediatric visit, I watched Andie's doctor fill out her growth chart—she was in the 75th percentile for weight and 90th percentile for height.

"Should we mail her old pediatrician a copy?" I asked Lee on my way home. "Ask if he can still pick out the preemie?"

Andie wears skinny jeans now, makes up dances behind her closed bedroom door, has contact lenses, and won't wear skirts to school because she complains that she can't run as fast as the boys. She reads Greek myths, plays the cello, and wants to learn Chinese, Spanish, and Latin (in addition to the German and French she's already learning in school). She fills the bird feeders in our yard, drinks herbal tea with honey, worries about global warming, and charges Lee and me a dollar every time we swear.

A friend recently asked her if she remembers anything from her time in the NICU. After some thought she replied, "Not really. Just a humming sound, like a vibration."

Before soccer games and ski races, Lee brushes Andie's long, blond hair into a ponytail and the two of them still occasionally flop on the floor for a game of "tickle monster."

From time to time I find him gazing at her. "She's just so beautiful," he says.

Tucker, now 13, is still Andie's greatest champion, and challenger. They recently came flying down a dual slalom ski course, trying to beat each other to the finish. "Just once you'd think he'd let her win," I said to a friend. "Are you kidding?" My friend laughed. "Getting beat by her is probably his greatest fear." And I realized he was right. Tucker has known Andie's potential all along.

Andie often touches her scars, wanting the stories repeated again and again. "Should I look into plastic surgery?" Lee asks her. "We can get them fixed." For now, she says no. "I kind of like them," she tells him. "They're a part of me."

My scars from Andie's birth are still a part of me, too. Although there are days when I actually forget they're there, I still have moments of panic when I fear another shoe will drop and everything will be lost. Then the kids remind me, "Breathe, Mom." And I do. I still marvel at the miracle of Andie's birth, but I've come to see that every birth is a miracle.

Last week the kids had the chance to go to a ski race on a Friday. "No way," Andie said. "I'm not missing school."

"What is *wrong* with you, Andie?" Tucker asked.

Andie shrugged. "That's just the kind of person I am."

And so she is. And I can't wait to see the person she continues to become.

ACKNOWLEDGMENTS

IF IT TAKES A VILLAGE to raise a child, I now know the same holds true for a book. And there is a village of people I wish to thank.

Thanks to my parents, who have always believed in me, often more than I've believed in myself.

Thanks to Lee's parents, whose quiet, constant love and support is not mentioned nearly enough within these pages.

To Libbie and Chris, John and Lollie, and Elizabeth and Todd. Lee and I won the lottery when it came to siblings and the spouses they chose.

Thanks to my aunts Mimi and Harriet, who are always just a phone call and care package away.

Thanks to my cousin Peter Kray, who not only hand delivered my husband, but offered a crash course in all things book publishing.

To our dear friends in Holliston, who gathered around and held us like family—and we thought we were just buying a house.

Special thanks to Pam and Tom Pendleton, who let us wear a foot path to their back door; Stephanie Danforth, who willingly became our 24/7 on-call nurse during those first few rough years; Nancy Galiardi, for letting me cry and heal in the back of her yoga studio; Karen Thalmann, whose life lessons provided perspective for my own; Leslie Rich, who ensured three months of dinner without dishes; Holly and Fletcher Wilson, who walked their own path of emotional challenges and found room to help us with ours; and Sandy Leverence, who literally baby-sat me from the beginning.

To Andie's nurses—Marcia, Tina, Yvonne, and Janice—and the entire staff at Brigham Women's and Children's Hospitals.

Thanks to Karen McCarthy, the glue that kept us together and made us whole again, and to Dawn Parker, who probably knew about this book long before I did!

To our devoted friends for their tireless belief in Andie *and* the book: Charlotte Gilet, Rob Ingall, Shandy Welch, Scarlett Plavocos, Rachael Rhine, Alison Shoemaker, Joe Keefe, Scott and Laura Beebe, Lucy McBride, and Molly Brandt.

To the incredible women in the Wilton Center Book Group, the Spirit Book Group, and The Writing Group (that still remains nameless!).

Thanks to the Pine Hill Waldorf community for nurturing and loving our children, and Kripalu Yoga Center where many of these words found their way to the page.

To Enid Ames, a treasured friend; Eleanor Owen, the southern sister I never knew I had; and Libby Barnett, my fairy Godmother.

I found many mentors along the way who were willing to share their time, expertise, and passion for writing: Sy Montgomery, Katrina Kenison, Steve Lewers, Nancy Mellon, Kim Ponders, Jeremy Townsend, Sue Hall, Renee Schuls-Jacobson, and Ramsay Thomas.

To Sue Ludwig of the National Association of Neonatal Therapists, your early support helped me believe in this book. And to Kelli Kelley of Hand to Hold, the organization she built from the ground up, providing peer-to-peer support to parents of preemies, babies born with special health care needs, and those who have experienced loss (www.handtohold.org).

To Suzanne Kingsbury, friend, editor, and writing coach extraordinaire. Just when I thought I couldn't dig any deeper, you pushed me even further to bring this story more fully to life. Thank you for your generous spirit and for sharing your remarkable talent.

To Dede Cummings, my fearless and passionate agent who became both the book's champion and guardian. I am awed by the energy, joy, and zeal you bring to every project you touch, including mine. Thank you for welcoming me into your magic circle.

Thanks also to Random House and the incredible crew at Hatherleigh Press: Andrew Flach, Ryan Tumambing, and Anna Krusinski, who live and breathe their inspiring mission statement. To Anna, I send my deepest gratitude for your brilliant editing skills.

To Andie, Tucker, and Lee, I'm so blessed to be on this team. Thank you for letting me share our story.

And finally, to all the babies and families who preceded us, your stories and contributions have shaped our outcome. We remain forever grateful.